BALANCE!

BALANCE!

A Handbook for Unsteady Seniors

By an Unsteady Senior
CHARLES PRESS

&

An Experienced Physical Therapist
DONALD H. BLOUGH

To order additional copies of this book, contact:
Xlibris LLC
1-888-795-4274
www.Xlibris.com
Orders@Xlibris.com
135178

Unsteady As a Senior?

BALANCE! A HANDBOOK FOR UNSTEADY SENIORS

DESIGNED TO HELP WITH YOUR PROBLEM

Our goal for unsteady Seniors is a modest one: to remain active while sharply reducing the probability of falling.

An unsteady Senior describes his experiences and discoveries and expresses opinions about both.

An experienced physical therapist briefly outlines the theory of balance and recommends exercises tailored for unsteady Seniors.

Eight unsteady Seniors from varied backgrounds plus the coauthor, show how to do the exercises (rather than svelte twenty-year-old young athletes in tights).

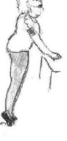

The unsteady Senior discusses facing up to the fear of falling (not forcing oneself to act bravely but only standing up and be willing to try a step or more). He suggests that the real risks are not the major hazards (like crawling around on roofs) but small risks we are all tempted to take, things that we used to do so easily.

No wonder we get impatient and take chances. He tells about downers, when what should not have happened did, describing a few falls he has taken, and analyzes why they happened (foolishness and blocked vision) and how they could have been prevented. He gives tips on what he found out doing the exercises and what he learned about keeping at it, preventing boredom and navigating safely.

Expertise to the rescue. The coauthor received his certification in Physical Therapy in Minnesota at the Mayo Clinic and has forty-four years experience in the field including heading a physical therapy center.

He recommends exercises specifically chosen for unsteady Seniors, describes the importance of posture, how to do stretches, strengthening and balance training, and exercises to correct walking problems, and discusses the art of falling and getting up.

Checking each other. Each author carefully reviewed and questioned the other's sections: the physical therapist, to make sure what was written was accurate, and the unsteady senior, to make sure all his questions were being answered.

Other features. We describe hopeful scientific research on balance, such as the BrainPort and bionic shoe vibrations, and review proposed aid from practitioners from acupuncture to ART and muscle activation techniques. We go over the Yale research on who is most likely to fall. We include the usual chapter about hazards around the house but note that, while most falls occur there, it's because that's where we, retired Seniors, spend much of our time. Most have corrected the obvious hazards, but we list them anyway.

Reference. We have chapters on supports: canes and braces and on how to treat common injuries and the medications available. The handbook concludes with a glossary of common terms.

Also, the word "Seniors" is capitalized throughout. And it's about time too!

To Nance, Melanie,

and absent friends.

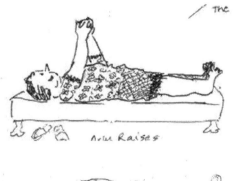

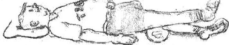

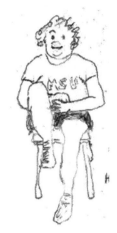

Seniors of all kinds

from all walks of life

may become unsteady.

Look closely at the next page. You will see a variety of types among our dream team of unsteady Senior exercisers—all retirees and all finding themselves now a little unsteady.

Begin with the woman with the cane and go clockwise. Barbara is a former school teacher whose left leg was injured in an auto accident. Next is Sam, who was an official at Michigan National Bank. Mildred is the wife of the retired minister at the United Methodist Church. Next is Lou, one of the MSU's star basketball players who came back as an assistant coach after his playing days in the NBA were over.

Ruthie stayed home taking care of her parents and after her mother died, began to make some needed extra cash as a cleaning lady. Then there's Pat, the big Irish former foreman at what used to be the Olds GM plant. Old-timer Pete, who comes next, just turned up then Clara, the wife of one of the most successful attorneys in the town's most established and prestigious law firm.

And there's also a stranger who somehow got into one of the exercise pictures. He's not shown here.

And also joining in the fun will be the coauthor of this handbook.

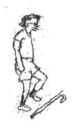
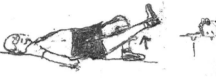

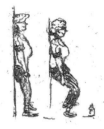
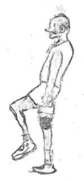

THE
SENIOR
EXERCISE
DREAM
TEAM

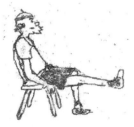

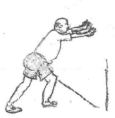
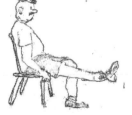

About the Authors

To begin with, we want to tell you a little about us—a kind of brief resume of our qualifications, as an unsteady Senior and as a physical therapist.

From the Unsteady Senior

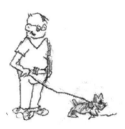 My name is Charlie Press, a semiretired Senior if we count hobbies. I served overseas in the U.S. Army, attended Elmhurst (Illinois) College and later on the GI Bill, the University of Missouri, and the University of Minnesota.

As a professor at Michigan State University, my job included writing some college text books filled with fascinating facts about Federalism and the separation of powers. Even then, I had latched on to a topic that had to do with a delicate balance, the checks on our presidents, courts and congress, checks that the founders thoughtfully embedded into our great U.S. Constitution to keep our nation steady.

Just like many of you, I gradually discovered I was an unsteady Senior. So, in my section of this handbook, you will get a rundown on the experiences and discoveries of someone struggling with our common problem. On the way, I have learned more useful facts about balance than I ever knew existed. From Don, I learned how to do exercises properly. It has helped me change the way I exercise and how I get around. And you will be surprised as I was to learn about the exciting research going forward about the balance problems of us Seniors.

While I'm not a bowler like my partner, Don, (He belongs to four bowling leagues!) I keep busy. My wife, Nance, and I used to take trips to Europe and Canada before the bottom dropped out of the dollar and air fares broke through the ceiling. So now it's Chicago and other USA locales, and Amtrak is the way to go.

Almost every day, Nance and I walk around the neighborhood with Dundee, our dog. In the summer, we walk a mile or so at our cottage on Lake Michigan. In the winter, I prefer to walk at the mall. The result is, I feel more stable and in less danger of falling; that is if I use common sense and follow other sensible suggestions found in this handbook.

The other day, the light on our garage door opener went out. It stayed out for about a week until we had friends over. Then out came the step ladder, and my buddy Gary fixed it with a few twists of one of those corkscrew bulbs that are supposed to last for seven years. Like most of you, I don't do step ladders anymore.

It's time that we, Seniors, faced up to the unfortunate fact that somehow we have arrived at being grown-ups. We don't expect to come across salves that will sprout a bushy head of hair overnight, and we become suspicious of "miracle cures."

So maybe you're a little disappointed that you don't find me claiming to do handsprings down our front driveway or entering bungee jumping contests.

Our recipe for recovery for me and other unsteady Seniors is a modest one—to remain active while sharply reducing the probability of falling. That's enough because it allows me to lead a pleasant Senior lifestyle, being wise enough to know that at our age, and into the future, just keeping what we have is a worthy goal.

But we also expect a little measurable progress as well when we put in a little effort. The medical researchers say this is what we can expect by following the kind of balance suggestions found in this handbook.

The doctors say unsteadiness is not inevitable for Seniors and that, with activity, we will keep or improve our balance. And this I have found to be the case.

Before ending, I want to thank my wife, Nance, who read my part of this handbook and approved of most of it.

FROM THE EXPERIENCED PHYSICAL THERAPIST

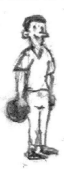

My name is Don Blough. At sixty-eight years, I am considered a Senior at many well-known establishments and organizations such as McDonald's, AARP and the United States Bowling Congress. I have been a practicing physical therapist for forty-four years.

My journey from Happy Meals to Senior coffee extended from Pennsylvania, with an undergraduate degree from Slippery Rock State College in Health and Physical Education in 1967, and thru to Minnesota for certification in Physical Therapy from the Mayo Clinic in 1969. Most of my career was spent in Michigan until a recent move to Georgia, where, in my retirement, I returned to full-time employment.

As a physical therapist, I was no respecter of age. Patient ages ranged from a few weeks to many well into their 90s. Likewise, there was no lack in the variety of ailments I was exposed to that involved balance problems such as stroke, multiple sclerosis, cancer, pulmonary dysfunctions, vestibular disturbances, and TMJ disorders as well as an assortment of orthopedic conditions and sports injuries, to name a few.

Notable clients have included Magic Johnson, professional basketball player, Clarence "Biggy" Munn, Michigan State University football coach, the Sheik, professional wrestler, and Bobby Unger, race car driver (and also Charlie).

Consultation opportunities over the years have utilized my expertise in areas far beyond my expectations. My testimony in front of an administrative court judge on barrier-free design, in part, paved the way for the first outdoor water slide in the State of Michigan. I was on the advisory boards for the Association of Shared Childbirth and for the Psychological Evaluation and Treatment Center. As a gymnast's father and as a member of the board of directors of Great Lakes Gymnastic Club, I had opportunities to evaluate and to modify conditioning techniques.

My expert opinions and testimonies were utilized by insurance companies, legal firms, and the state's attorney general's office. The undergraduate teacher's training I received was put to good use in my capacity as a clinical instructor, as a speaker at the Michigan State's Sports Medicine Interest Group, as a presenter to adult-enhancement programs, and as a guest professor to the Michigan State University, Osteopathic undergraduate medical students.

"Therapeutic Insights" was my business in my brief retirement and best describes what I did. The therapeutic insights for this handbook come from years of formal education, well enhanced by a blend of personal and professional experience gleaned from both junior and Senior perspectives.

A successful rehab program is dependent upon a well-defined approach specific to each of your situations and one that is faithfully pursued. However, failure to fulfill personal expectations may not be for a lack of effort but may be due to the varied and complex nature of your condition. For many, positive results will be realized within days or weeks, while others' progress will be accomplished in months or even perhaps in a slower regression in balance and function.

What you can expect to get out of this handbook is the opportunity to become adept at determining what works for you. Many options will be presented and your responsibility is to find which ones will be beneficial.

As a reminder, this is not a line dance where everybody does the same footwork. This is life where sometimes you are the only person in step with the music, or so it seems.

Become an expert in *you* since you're the one person with *you* most, day and night.

Also, be flexible in your thinking. Know when to vary the program both in intensity as well as in techniques.

To improve is to change. To become closer to perfect is to change often.

CONTENTS

PART THREE
A Reference File of Useful Information

PART FOUR

An Overview of What's Ahead

What you have in your hands is a handbook of not one but three interconnecting and interrelated parts.

Part One: The Unsteady Senior Part

The first section is about my (Charlie) experiences in search of enlightenment and improvement in balance.

You will find what I discovered in checking what the researchers claimed would help and why. This includes studies about which Seniors are most likely to fall, the latest research on unsteadiness that is going forward, and information about the variety of techniques practitioners offer, from massage and Tai Chi to acupuncture and imaging.

You will also find that I describe some of my own falls and why they happened as well as things I have learned through experience about exercising and navigating and in keeping at it without getting bored.

Part Two: The Physical Therapy Part

I (Don) discuss what physical therapists know and recommend about exercise for unsteady Seniors, types of equipment, and places where you may exercise—in physical therapy, health clubs, or at home.

The self tests I recommend allow each unsteady Senior to discover his or her own specific weaknesses and plan a program to address them. The tests also set markers unsteady Seniors can check on their progress.

Then I outline a step-by-step program for attacking the balance difficulties of unsteady Seniors, including correcting problems Seniors may have in walking.

PART THREE: THE REFERENCE PART

This section puts together facts that we unsteady Seniors may not want to memorize but have available in a format easy to reference.

You will find what to do in the case of a serious injury as well as for those injuries that are less serious but still painful such as strains, sprains, or muscle cramps.

You will find out what the researchers say about supports from analgesics to braces and their best advice on getting canes and walkers. There's even a brief discussion about how to interpret those ever-present research findings we come across reported in newspapers and magazines.

And we end with a glossary of terms commonly used by physicians, trainers, and physical therapists.

INTERCONNECTIONS

I, Charlie, (the unsteady Senior) wanted to be sure that Don, the physical therapist, answered the questions we unsteady Seniors want answered. I, Don, (the physical therapist) wanted to be sure the information in the chapters that Charlie, the unsteady Senior, wrote didn't wander off the reservation. So each us reviewed the other's chapters in detail. After a little fine tuning, both of us ended up happy with the other's chapters as well as our own, and we think, so will you.

A WORD ABOUT STYLE

We use the term *"Seniors"* to describe those over sixty-five. Some suggest other laudatory terms such as the Seasoned or the Sages or maybe even the Whoopee Geezers. But we suggest that we'd better not go tinkering, or, the next thing we know, those Senior Tuesdays at the groceries will disappear and we'll be paying full price for everything.

You will also find that grand word *"Senior"* is consistently capitalized throughout and it's about time. As far as we have come, we deserve a little respect.

We know how Casey Stengel felt after a successful career as manager of the New York Yankees. But when he reached age seventy, he was fired. The front office said they wanted to put in a youth program. He said he learned a big lesson. "I'll never make the mistake of being seventy years old again."

But Casey Stengel went on to new triumphs, winning pennants as manager of several other major league teams and ended up in the Baseball Hall of Fame in Cooperstown.

Success with your unsteadiness also lies ahead for you.

So there you have it.

If you are a Senior faced with a balance situation, in this Handbook, you will find the most comprehensive collection of up-to-date, reliable information and recommendations about improvement for unsteadiness.

Cheers!

PART ONE

A PILGRIM'S PROGRESS

(from very unsteady to less unsteady Senior)
And what he learned along the way
about balancing

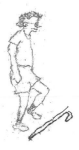 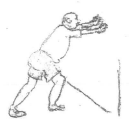

Chapter 1

HAVING A BALANCE PROBLEM

When you read a *"we"* in this section, it isn't some twenty-two-year-old receptionist welcoming one of us Seniors into the doctor's office with "Hi, honey" or "Hi, darlin'" or "Hi, sweetie" or maybe "Hi, Henrietta" or "Hi, Herbert" as if we Seniors were all children. And then she adds, "How are *we* feeling today?"

In what follows, *"we"* means all of us Seniors with balance problems, including me, Charlie.

Let's be honest about this unsteadiness thing right from the start. This Senior is still a work in progress. Not only have I been there, I'm still working around and in and out of that big unsteadiness neighborhood.

Plenty of experts are out there, shouting out helpful directions at us Seniors, how we should be building up our muscles, etc. They're worth listening to, but later on, when we tackle an exercise, they're not where we are, down on the floor with us, some miles away to be sure but also doing one of those same old stretchers.

When you do a proprioception—(I just put it in to call your attention to the glossary in the reference chapter 43. I promise, from now on, I won't give you any more gymnastic jaw-breakers standing alone.) As I was saying, when you're doing one of those balance positioning exercises to get an idea fixed in your head about where your feet go to, you can picture me also awkwardly kicking out one of my legs and also wondering where it goes.

WE'RE ALL CANDIDATES FOR A FALL

The Centers for Disease Control and Prevention recently reported that a greater number of Seniors are having more falls than just fifteen years ago. They say it's because there are more of us, and we are living longer and so are more likely have vision loss and loss of muscle strength.

The American Academy of Orthopedic Surgeons says falls are the leading cause of injuries for Americans over sixty-five. Fortunately, only one in ten or so of these falls result in a serious injury, but that's bad enough. (Don has a chapter on how to fall and lessen the chances of getting hurt.)

You can skip the next paragraph if you don't want to read again the gruesome details about falls.

More than 1.5 million Seniors are treated in emergency rooms each year, and 400,000 are hospitalized because of falls. And an estimated 10,000 Americans over sixty-five, they say, die each year from injuries related to serious falls. One-fourth of those with broken hips die within a year. Half are never able to walk again without a cane or walker. Forty percent never return to their own homes again but go to a nursing home or live with relatives.

My balance situation. Like many of us Seniors with a balance problem, I, too, have been a first-class candidate for a fall. As the result, in an earlier life of chasing little rubber balls with a racket, and occasionally getting whacked somewhere, I have had to take part in three knee replacement operations because arthritis had then eaten away my knee cartilage. That number is right; after a couple of years, the plastic insert in one of the knee replacements broke, and I went through it again.

When I began this handbook, I had some infuriating falls that I'll describe later on.

Still I get around using a cane whenever I anticipate trouble, especially when I go to a movie or play and think I may have to go up and down steps without those friendly railings or when I go into one of those romantically, darkened restaurants. Keeping a cane in the car, I've found, is a good idea.

Never have I met a handrail I didn't like. And towel racks too, sometimes, but only to touch, not to hold me up. And I've found that walls are good friends.

In summer, as I walk the Lake Michigan roads, my wife, Nance, a demon walker—for her age—is usually far ahead, but she's humane. In the past, she sometimes said she was tempted to write a piece, "Seeing the Sights with the Kids, Twenty Feet behind Charlie Press," but it's all different now. I've slowed down. When Nance gets too far ahead, she walks in little circles until I catch up. But you can cheat a little by crouching down, loping along like Groucho Marx. Try it if you doubt me.

You can get a demonstration of this technique in the bird-watching scene in the movie *Mr. Hobbs Takes a Vacation,* starring Jimmy Stewart and Maureen O'Hara. Those of us Seniors who have grown up kids will also find the rest of the movie an enjoyable "right on!" But hurry up and see it before Steve Martin does a remake.

So How Did I Get Into Writing This Handbook?

Let me tell you my sad story.

Some years ago, I began to notice that sometimes I was off balance. Slowly, it got worse. For some time, I did very little about it, thinking that, by just walking around and doing a few exercises now and then, I'd get along okay.

One day, I read, while waiting in a grocery line, that I could improve my balance if I just stood on one foot for ten seconds or so. But I knew that if I tried that, I'd not only fall on my face, but I'd also scatter the display of those sensational scandal magazines all over the check-out counter and also probably take down one or two customers in line ahead of me.

I had to face up to it; I had a balance problem. Newscaster Bob Schieffer says a lesson he learned in his Texas boyhood was, "When you have to, you will." When I finally realized what I had to, I decided I would try to do something about my balance situation.

What I did. In the Beginning, I began observing myself more closely. Maybe like you, I began to look at my reflection in shop windows as I walked along to see if I could figure out what I might be doing wrong. At the mall, I watched how others walked—those in trouble and those not. When I walked around in my socks, which I later found was a no-no, I noticed that my left sock was the one that always ended up flapping.

Looking at my footprints in the sand, I noticed I took shorter steps with my left foot. Also, I could see that Nance's footprints showed that she pushed off with her toes while mine just made a deep indentation with my heel and no evidence of push off.

When I tried to keep in step with some Seniors ahead of me in a mall, I noticed I had to speed up. Try it and you may be a little surprised as I was. But don't get too close, or you may get in trouble for stalking.

When Don read over this section, he strongly seconded the idea of watching your own actions; however, he also suggested asking others to observe us as we walk or exercise and to report their findings. Spouses and friends may be holding back helpful suggestions out of a sense of good manners.

Nance, one day, did tell me that I was bending over as I walked. I hadn't really noticed. So I tried straightening up, shoulders back, head up, back straight, and lifting thine eyes unto the mountains or anyhow look straight ahead. The effect was amazing.

You know, I seemed to walk better, and I began seeing things I never noticed before, nothing of great importance but still. And I kid you not; it kind of gave me a happy lift.

So how did I exercise? Like most of us Seniors with balance situations, I had let my muscles get a little flabby, and my range of motion could perhaps be improved; that is through carrying out arm and leg movements to the fullest extent. And I noticed that once or twice I stumbled, not being exactly sure where all my feet had gone.

For a long time, I went about this pretty haphazardly. To get those exercises exactly right didn't seem important. Later, I found out why those fussy physical therapists, like Don, seemed to think differently.

On some days, I forgot to exercise, which happens, but mostly I kept trying. None of us is perfect or wants to be. As helter-skelter as this all was, it still seemed to me that after a while, I sensed some improvement.

Getting helpful advice. At the same time, I began trying to find out more about unsteadiness.

Unsteady Seniors told me about their experiences. Here's a tip that one who's been there told me. When you feel a little wobbly, whether sitting or standing, you should stop and focus on something vertical such as a tree trunk or telephone pole.

And I asked experts my questions, when I thought of them, which sometimes occurred to me too late. Four times, I had been in physical therapy—once after arthroscopic surgery, which was a couple years before my first knee replacement and then three times after each.

That's, as I've already said, how I had first met Don Blough, physical therapist par excellence.

The physical therapists gave me some of the answers that helped fill in some of the blanks. They all suggested exercises that would help. But in time I tended to forget their advice and mislay what they had written down for me.

Some friends told me their doctors fob them off when they raise the topic of unsteadiness with phrases like "Well now, consider your age . . ."

That's not been my experience. Mine have been most helpful with suggestions and answering my questions, stupid no not.[1]

Searching out printed information. I also began to look for whatever I could find on this vital topic. I clipped newspaper stories and magazine articles and checked the internet. Back then, I found very few articles on balance itself, though this began to change. My pile of clippings and torn out magazine articles began to grow like

---

[1] Would you mind if I thank them personally here: my primary physicians, Dr. Marlene Harvey and when she retired, Dr Sreenivasa Murthy of Blue Care Network of Michigan, the orthopod who did my knee surgeries, Dr. Edward Sladek, and Dr. Glen Ackerman, neurologist and also a personal friend, Dr. Joseph Vorro, Michigan State University Family and Community Medicine, who gave me encouragement and suggestions. Don would also like to thank Dr. Sladek who took it upon himself to know the physical therapists to whom he sent his patients, having the confidence that quality care would be provided consistent with his protocols.

Mopsie, our baby kitten, now a cat. That cutesy name didn't come from me—Troubles is a better fit. But she's grown up to be a pesky but loveable feline who wants to stay out all night if we'd just let her.

A study in Britain, that I came across, (reported in the November 2007 issue of the *Journal of the American Geriatrics Society*) says that Seniors who get into an exercise program can protect themselves against the loss of ability to walk, climb stairs, maintain a sense of balance, and sustain grip strength. What more could we ask for?

My file folder full of unsorted data got fatter and fatter. Exercises were being suggested everywhere but not always with unsteady Seniors in mind.

The search for a handbook on balance. But there were gaps.

Surely, I thought, all this information about balance must be gathered together handy in one place somewhere. Exercise books were flooding the bookstores. And so I looked hard and long for one that dealt specifically with balance for us Seniors and found not one.

With mounting irritation, I browsed through what was there, looking in the indexes under "balance." At most, I found only a short paragraph or two; most authors changed the subject quickly after recommending Tai Chi and Yoga.

In one of the many books available, I did find a long section devoted to balance. So I bought the book and began to read.

There were balance exercises all right. The book advised healthy young athletes that they should get actively involved in "Dynamic Balance Training," (that, for example, is when another baseball player slides into you while you're playing second base as you try to keep your balance for a throw to first). If you succeed, you are balanced dynamically, I guess.

These techniques could no doubt sharpen athletic performance in all sorts of strenuous contact sports. All we had to do was follow some exhausting acrobatic drills involving bongo and wobble boards. Since long ago, I gave up my ambition to play third base for the St. Louis Cardinals; I found this book only partially helpful. Still, it was not a total loss.

A handbook on Balance for Seniors, I concluded, was desperately needed, and I bravely decided I would try to write one.

Stepping stones toward recovery. Missouri, where I grew up, is called the Show-me state, and I suppose that's why I wanted to know the "why" behind what the experts said would help us unsteady Seniors. Why would it help? The answer had to be grounded in reliable research findings such as those published in reputable medical and professional journals. And when I tried it on me, it had to work.

Before I accepted the recommendations of any expert, I wanted to be sure they didn't come out of thin air. When I found something useful, I called it a stepping stone to recovery.

My definition for recovery has been a relatively modest one—it is staying active while sharply reducing the probability of falling.

And so I began writing this Handbook.

After I had gotten a good start, Nance stepped in with some good wifely advice. She gently pointed out that I was not an authority on everything and especially on what other people, with different problems, should do to help themselves. For that, I needed an expert in the field to back me up and check me.

Almost immediately, I remembered Don, my former physical therapist. He agreed to work with me, and a really helpful handbook became a possibility.

Meanwhile I began to change my ways. Now, I began to exercise more carefully and in a more structured program and took more seriously what the experts said. I can't tell you how many times this has made me go back and reread sections of Don's chapters. I achieved, overtime, the kind of balance that was second nature when I was in my twenties, thirties, forties, and so on? Are you kidding? As yet, I have found no secret miracle cures to pass on. My goal has been measurable progress.

But as we Seniors know, sometimes just keeping what we have and for some, maybe even slowing down the decline, is measurable progress. I'm still not where I'd like to be. Unfortunately, it's not a perfect world. But, I'm also not where I once was. And that's something.

In all honesty, I should also add that signs of improvement sometimes took longer to come than I expected.

But as one physical therapist once said to me with some tartness, "Look, it took you ten years or more to get into this shape; why do you think you can get back to your old form in just a couple weeks?"

Nevertheless, I steadily improved. The times between falls were getting much longer. At one point back when I first noticed this, I bragged to myself that I couldn't even remember the last time that I fell, which was true. But that fellow who wrote "pride goeth before the fall" knew what he was talking about. Not long after, boom, and down I went.

When someone asks me now if I've fallen recently, I just answer, "Not Yet." This is because we can never know what we might meet out there in the big wide world—maybe a skateboarder or someone behind us in a hurry to get through a revolving door. Or we forget and turn suddenly or reach for something too far away. Or we may just do something really stupid and think we can get away with it. Still, I usually go for many, many months without even coming close to a fall.

So there's hope ahead for all of us unsteady Seniors. You may improve a good deal faster than I have.

You are probably in better shape than I was.

The next step. Before describing my stepping stones to recovery, I'm going to suggest that, in the next couple chapters, it might be helpful in keeping our spirits high for us to get an overview of what's going on out there to help us unsteady Seniors—the experiments the researchers are making and all the therapies devised by practitioners to make life easier for us unsteady Seniors.

On the other hand, you may want to just dip in to each of the next two chapters and put them aside for later and move right on to Chapter 4 on page 53, which tells who the researchers at Yale Program on Aging found to be the Seniors most likely to fall.

AN UNSTEADY SENIOR FACES UP TO HAVING A BALANCE PROBLEM WHAT WAS THAT CHAPTER ALL ABOUT?

We unsteady Seniors are all works in progress, all candidates for a fall. I first tried on my own to improve and then looked around for some reliable help. I found out that researchers say we can improve. But no handbook thus far exists that gathers in one handy place all the information about balance for Seniors and gives us expert guidance from an established physical therapist as well as what we unsteady Seniors have learned on our own.

This handbook aims to fill that gap.

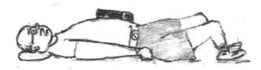

Chapter 2

THE UNSTEADY SENIOR DISCOVERS
THE HOPEFUL RESEARCH GOING ON

Donna Shalala, former secretary of health and human services said it, and she got it precisely right.

"There *never* has been a better time to be older than today."

The experts in many fields are now paying attention to the problems of us Seniors, including our balance problems. A great deal of help is now out there, and more is on the way.

Just think back to the kind of world your parents and grandparents lived in. About the only exercises were the Daily Dozen developed mainly for soldiers in World War I, and most people had never heard of them. Gym classes in schools were often a joke, especially for women. Few people talked seriously about obesity or the problems of unsteadiness.

The only ones interested in exercise and diet were a few professional athletes and those characters other people dismissed as "health nuts." People assumed bad things like unsteadiness just happened to people, and that's the way it was and always would be, and there wasn't much you could do about it.

As you read the descriptions of the research going on, I think you will be impressed. The distance between pure research and its practical application is very small indeed and getting smaller.

THE CUTTING EDGE OF RESEARCH ON BALANCE FOR SENIORS

Sensors and nerves. The current research on balance is on our communication system—the dulling of sensors or receptors, especially at the bottom of our feet. This is a major way we get the messages that help us control our movements. Attention is also is being paid to the decline in effectiveness of the nerves that carry the balance messages up to the brain and send back directions.

The goal is to make this communication system as efficient as the one when we start to pick up a hot dish. Then the brain flashes back a message immediately to move our fingers to a more pleasant location. We lack similar messages about where our feet are.

Retraining our brains. The researchers say we can also start at the brain end of the communication system to build up what they call position sense. They say we have allowed the stored images in our cerebellums to fade. We can reinvigorate old images or create new brain images of where our feet and hands are—what physical therapists call muscle memory.

Another part of retraining our brain is called imaging or visualization. Those treating very serious injuries have found just imaging recovering use of limbs helps the injured. Just thinking can sometimes make it so.

Getting back muscle strength. Yet even if we regain accurate messages from those sensors and also recreate position sense, we may still be wobbly if our leg and muscles are so weak and stiff.

At one time, people just exercised without much thought about the effects of particular exercises. They just hoped it would help. Now, physical therapists, athletic trainers, and others, have been examining more closely what each exercise can accomplish and how it may be best done. They don't go along hit-and-miss but target exercises to correct specific problems. And, overall, the goal is to retain or bring back muscle strength.

RETRAINING THOSE INACTIVE SENSORS AND NERVES

This emphasis is on rejuvenating sensors, especially those receptors found on the soles of our feet.

Bionic shoe vibrations. Dr. Jim Collins, a professor of Bioengineering at Boston University, has experimented with bionic shoes, socks, and insoles that create randomized, fluctuating, weak vibrations, what the scientists whimsically call noise. These, he had found, wake up those lackadaisical receptors. Three battery-powered elements are embedded in elastic silicone gel to create the vibrations.

Dr. Collins claims, "The vibrations enabled seventy-five-year-olds to balance as well as twenty-three-year-olds." They were able to stand quietly without swaying or losing their balance.

All this is still in the experimental stage, but we unsteady Seniors can be sure that such products might turn up one of these days in an ad in the AARP magazine and perhaps at a reasonable price.

The biaxial body energizer. The Journal of the American Academy of Neurology, Neurology Now (May/June 2006) reports clinical trials are going forward on a procedure using magnets to stimulate sensors and nerves. Dr. Michael Weintraub, MD, clinical professor of Neurology at New York medical College in Valhalla, NY, became interested in the power of magnets after several patients reported they relieved pain. He had fourteen patients wear magnetized insoles even while asleep. After four months, he found that nerve conduction improved with a decrease in feelings of numbness. He then conducted a more rigorous double-blind study, in which the patients were unaware of whether they received the treatment or a placebo. He got similar results.

Next, he developed an apparatus that looks like a bathroom scale and has twirling magnets. It is to be used two hours a day for ninety days. This is now being tested on 250 volunteers at fifteen university diabetic centers and ten private medical groups across the country.

REPAIRING THE COMMUNICATION SYSTEM

The research and experiments on the nerves that communicate have been aimed primarily at those who are paralyzed from a spinal injury. But they potentially also have relevance for us unsteady Seniors who are not getting accurate messages.

FES (Functional Electrical Stimulation) Therapy. Dr. John W. McDonald of Baltimore's Kennedy Krieger Institute, the doctor for "Superman" star Christopher Reeves, developed a therapy involving bicycles with sticky pads that give electrical jolts to leg muscles. These shocks are supposed to stimulate the leg muscles to push the pedals.

The electrical jolts are aimed at nerves in the spine that had become dormant. The electricity, he says, not only stimulates these nerves but, at the same time, causes the brain to store bicycling patterns of motion. The procedure was designed to teach the nerves to carry signals to the arms and legs and might even form new connections.

Muscle regeneration after a spinal injury generally occurs naturally in the first six months, if at all, and never after the first year and a half. Researchers using this electric shock procedure caused Christopher Reeves to regain the ability to feel, touch, and move his feet more than five years later, and that's considered very unusual.

In 2002, Dr. McDonald published a report in a medical journal of his further experiments with forty-eight paralyzed adults. Since then, seventy or so rehab centers are using FES cycling therapy. Dr. Randal Betz of Philadelphia Shriners Hospital for Children is conducting a rigorous study of FES therapy with thirty children aged 5 to 13.

Creating new neuronal pathways. Researchers hypothesized that within the spinal cord are pattern generators. These generators do not need to receive messages from the brain but when stimulated, can control muscles and send messages back to the brain. The procedure uses whatever a patient has left after a spinal injury.

Using a Lokomat, a robotically-assisted rehabilitation device that holds an injured person up on a treadmill with a series of straps, researchers at the Christopher and Dana Reeve Foundation were able to change one woman's life. A spinal injury from an auto accident left her paralyzed from the neck down with only a 1 percent prognosis of ever walking again. She took the treatment and after four months, was able to walk using crutches.

The researchers say they created new neuronal pathways. The Christopher and Dana Reeve Foundation has launched its NeuroRecovery Network that began locomotor training at seven hospitals.

You may think this is the far out cutting edge, but read on.

Nerve transplant. Some injuries cut a nerve and leave an arm or leg totally disabled. Dr. Susan Mackinnon, chief of plastic and reconstructive surgery at the School of Medicine at Washington University in St. Louis, has successfully transplanted a nerve from another part of the body across this gap. Perhaps, someday, techniques like this may be used to cover the gap between sensors in our feet to where the nerve going down the leg stops receiving signals. That's why I included it here.

Regenerative therapies. Now for the really far way out, check out what they're trying to do at the University of Pittsburgh McGowen Institute for Regenerative Medicine, Stanford University, and the University of California, San Francisco, as well as at other medical research centers. The injuries of wounded veterans have encouraged regenerative research efforts to attempt to have the body replace damaged nerves, fingers, or even limbs.

Scientists have observed that when a starfish loses a leg, it grows another back. Can scientists help the human body replace missing body parts? That's what they mean by regenerative research.

It began in the 1980s with the discovery that a substance in pigs' intestines could help grow human tissue. The studies are now on whether the substance can regenerate human fingers. Others are using electric field devices to stimulate regrowth in the spinal cord.

Some medical scientists are studying how to regenerate nerves and repair bones and ligaments. Using stem cell injections, the studies are concentrating on rejuvenating an injured heart muscle. Scientists have had some success in the growing of organs in the laboratory.

The bionic nervous system. Dr. John Donoghue, professor of Engineering and Neuroscience at Brown University, has developed a machine to bypass the nervous system altogether creating a bionic nervous system to replace it. A tiny sensor is implanted in the brain. This transmits thoughts as signals to a computer programmed to translate them into simple actions.

A paralyzed woman was able to direct a robotic arm to pick up a glass just through her thoughts. She had bypassed the break in her nervous system by using a bionic substitute. Could such a bionic substitute be used to solve the problem of peripheral neuropathy—not getting messages from sensors in the feet?

Biofeedback. This technique is included more as information than for the help it has thus far given us, unsteady Seniors. The theory is that the patient can be taught to control body functions based on the feedback of auditory or visual cues, perhaps rejuvenate the nervous communication system.

The patient is attached to a machine which sends signals—a flashing light or beeps. For stroke victims, the machine is attached to muscles and picks up electrical signals. The patient follows the flashing light or beeper that operates when the muscle is tensed. The patient then tries to relax the muscle. A clinician guides the process.

Those disabled by a stroke have been helped most. Since the late 1960s, biofeedback has been used successfully to treat stress and pain, and illnesses such as epilepsy and paralysis and other movement disorders. Success with the technique for balance problems has not been as great as was at first hoped. In a sense, nature has set limits on the level of improvement.

We Seniors can get further information from The Association for Applied Psychophysiology and Biofeedback (formerly the Biofeedback Society of America) at 1-800-477-8892 or 303-422-8436 or on the web at http//www.aapb.org. The association sponsors meetings and publishes a journal as well as other publications.

KLUTZINESS: RETRAINING OUR POSITION SENSE

This theory attacks the problem in what's going on upstairs. It concentrates on retraining the brain to better position sense. In the FES electrical experiments described above, you may have noticed that one of the results was causing certain bicycling patterns of motion for the brain to store.

The cerebellum, a clump of neurons in the back of the brain, is the area that has long been associated with balance and coordination and is where the memory storing takes place.

The researchers suggest we lose the physical memory of how our legs and feet behave—what the researchers call position sense or proprioception. And our memory of reflex actions also becomes blurred.

Research suggests that we can retrain our brain to strengthen our position sense by carefully repeating patterns of motion.

Balance exercises. The theory behind balance exercises is that we are retraining our brains by sending them precise movements to replace blurred images.

The balance exercises Don will detail later on are designed to give our brains this sense of where our feet are located at any time. Most can be done without special equipment.

Tai Chi (Tie Chee). Along with all the other stuff we import from China are a series of slow movements called Tai Chi, a big hope for those of us with the klutziness kind of balance problem. Researchers have found that those of us unsteady Seniors who do Tai Chi have better balance, probably because as we sway through the slow movements, getting them down precisely, we sense where our bodies are as we shift weight from one foot to the other.

Tai Chi involves postures and gestures given in sets or forms named after assorted Chinese creatures like lions and such. The series of slow, gentle, graceful moves are low impact; much like a ballet in slow motion. They help improve balance and coordination by reminding us how to shift weight from one foot to the other as we turn or step out. Some have called the process "swimming in air." They also improve our concentration—"meditation in motion."

One study found that a group of Seniors in their seventies, who were in Tai Chi for fifteen weeks, halved their risk of falling. Several other studies have confirmed these results.

The International Taoist Tai Chi Society lists instructors and classes at www.taoist.org, or you can look in the yellow pages under "Martial Arts," but get one that stresses relaxation and health.

Ballroom dancing. Researchers have found that doing the precise and repetitive movements of dancing will also help us improve our balance, again by making us aware of where our feet got to, though some of us, even in better days, never could seem to get the hang of always keeping off our partner's feet. If we don't have a partner handy, we can dance with a chair, a pillow, or a doll.

One experiment reported in the December 2007 issue of the *Journal of Neurologic Physical Therapy* found improvement in stretching, balance, footwork, and timing for Parkinson's patients who took twenty Tango lessons. The lead author was Madeleine E. Hackney of the Washington University School of Medicine in St. Louis.

The BrainPort device for balance. Professor Paul Bach-y-rita, a physician and neuroscientist at the University of Wisconsin, after watching his father's remarkable recovery from a stroke, theorized that our brains may be able to reorganize their functions in response to learning or experience. His theory suggests that if the message receptor from one of our senses breaks down, the brain can create another receptor to take over its function.

The scientists with the help of engineers designed the BrainPort, which, through a computer, sends signals on what to do to correct one's balance. If the subject lurches too far off balance in one direction, the computer sends a signal to bring him or her back upright.

Their first subject was a woman who lost her vestibular sense through a mistake in a prescription. After the first short treatment she regained her balance for a few minutes. Later treatments were lengthened to an hour, then to a day, and finally she was able to give up treatment altogether with her vestibular sense fully restored.

The group hopes to use the procedure on patients with Parkinson's disease and others with balance problems. Presently they are conducting clinical trials. They have also developed a treatment for the blind and have succeeded in getting them to see blurry moving images on a TV screen.

The technique of imaging or visualization. Physicians tell persons who have been completely immobilized, say by an auto accident, to imagine their recovery while still in bed unable to move. This means they imagine they are using the injured arms or legs just as they used to, thinking in pictures rather than words. They visualize themselves with everything working normally and expect it to happen. The practitioners call it "seeing your way well" or guided imagery. It sounds a little crazy, but my doctor friend tells me that it works, at least for the victims of auto accidents.

Many have argued that what we think influences action. Dr. Sam Maniar, a sports psychologist, demonstrated this by having a group of athletes each hold a piece of string with a washer tied to it. He then asked them to think about moving the washer from side to side without making the actual movement. To their amazement, in every case, the washer began to move. What was happening is that, without the athletes being aware of it, their brains were sending the message to the nerve receptors in their fingers to move the washer.

One experiment with imaging was at a weight loss resort. Exercisers who listened to imaging tapes that told them they were losing weight, lost twice the weight as exercisers who didn't.

Another experiment was with five stroke victims who watched videos with themselves superimposed into the action. They saw themselves diving with sharks, snowboarding down a narrow slope, and walking up a flight of stairs. Researchers reported they improved in walking, standing, and climbing steps better than a control group.

More intriguing, a brain scan showed a change in how their brains functioned. Note that the sample size was small, and researchers stressed that virtual reality experiments like this were only one of several types of interventions used with stroke victims.

Doing such imaging as we exercise can do no harm. As we go through the motions, we can visualize those sensors waking up and sending urgent messages for our nerves to get cracking and send signals up our legs and on to the spinal cord and then up to headquarters located above the neck. We unsteady Seniors can imagine ourselves back the way we were—playing volleyball, tap dancing, or even that our muscles are bulging like the Great Hulk.

One time we can do this is dreaming up some soothing thoughts as we drift off to sleep. We can hum a few bars of "Bright Winter Day, Calls Us Away" or "The Skaters Waltz" and imagine ourselves sailing in tandem with a fantasy companion across a deserted frozen lake. We can imagine ourselves dancing doing "The Nutcracker," going through those calming Tai Chi motions or imaging how to slip into our pants without holding on to something.

Dore Achievement Centers for Attention Deficit Disorder (ADD). This disorder was described in an article that caught my eye because it has relevancy for unsteady Seniors. The theory here is that ADD subjects need to do exercises of "cerebellar stimulation."

They balance on a wobble board, toss a bean bag from one hand to the other while sitting on a large Swiss plastic ball, and move their head from side to side while keeping their eyes on a fixed point.

RETRAINING THOSE CRAZY-LAZY MUSCLES

An English researcher, Jeremy N. Morris, back in 1949, nailed down the fact that exercise is good for everyone. He studied the conductors and drivers of those English double-decker buses and found that the conductors who were busy climbing the stairs and going inside to collect the fares were healthier and lived longer than the drivers who had to sit behind the wheel all day. Incidentally, Morris himself lived to be ninety-nine or as he insisted, plus a half.

Exercise for Seniors. Some of us Seniors remember how Jack LaLanne on his TV show tried to get us to exercise way back in the 1950s and beyond. He was still going strong at ninety-three, so maybe we should have listened more closely. To celebrate his ninety-fourth birthday, he planned to swim the twenty miles from the California coast to Catalina Island.

The Daily Dozen. During World War I, the famous football coach of the Yale champions, Walter Camp, worked out a series of exercises for privates, gobs, and civilians that he called the Daily Dozen." The writer P. G. Wodehouse did them every morning until he died at age ninety-two. But most Americans paid little attention once the war ended. The Daily Dozen, recommended by Camp, were intuitive but lacked a scientific basis. However, the people who did them got moving and just that alone helped.

Joseph H. Pilates exercises. In the 1980s, gymnasts began analyzing which exercises affected which muscles and how best to do them to achieve a desired result. Then they discovered the work of Joseph H. Pilates, a German gymnast and boxer who was in England teaching self defense to detectives, when World War I broke out. He was immediately interned and during the war had time in detention to sharpen his exercise program for himself and the other prisoners.

After the war, he opened exercise centers in Germany. In 1926, he came to the U.S. where he specialized in exercises designed for professional ballet dancers. He wrote several books, developed a set of thirty-four movements, and worked out over five hundred exercises. Many of the exercises we do today, except perhaps those we do for balance, can be traced back to his pioneering efforts. He died at age eighty-seven in 1967.

Pilates emphasized correct posture, correct spinal and pelvic alignment, precise form, proper breathing, and, above all, *control*. In fact, he called his system *Contrology* to stress the importance of making our minds watch closely what we are doing as we exercise. He emphasized intense concentration. He seemed to have thought of our minds as a muscle that also needed to be exercised.

The most important element of the Pilates exercise program was core strengthening the muscles he called the body's powerhouse. The core for Pilates was that band of about twenty-nine muscles that circle our torso at the hips, spinal, pelvic, and abdominal region. Strengthening these core muscles, he believed, would stabilize our spines and pelvis.

Also he believed that strong core muscles would lead to a better transfer of power to the extremities: our legs, arms, and shoulders. When a pitcher throws a ball, the power doesn't come only from his arm and shoulder as it would if he were standing still and throwing. It also comes from the leg, hip, abdomen, and back muscles, which transfer power generated in the core muscles outward. As kids, we boys used to call using only arm and maybe the shoulder to throw as "throwing like a girl." But not anymore! Women have caught up.

Pilates argued strengthening the core would lead to fewer injuries and would prevent lower back pain. Today, neurologists are suggesting that strong core muscles may also help with those balance problems.

Many variations of the Pilates core program have sprung up. Raebok has one that includes a set of exercises performed on the company's specially designed "core board."

Tailoring the exercise to the individual. In Oregon, *The Oregon Health and Science Research on Walking* had Senior volunteers equipped with sensors to study their walking and activity patterns. Some sensors were even embedded in the carpets. They measured precisely each person's walking speed, stride length, step width, and body sway to assess their risk of falling. These data were then used to decide which exercises would help each individual. In Ireland, *The Technology Research for Independent Living* completed a similar study of six hundred Seniors. They reported by tailoring the exercise to the individual they reduced falls by 30 percent.

Cross Training. One of the first discoveries that gymnasts made was that muscles need twenty-four hours to recover from strengthening exercises. Some suggest that as we grow older, a two-day wait between strengthening exercises is a good idea.

Physical therapists like Don recommend we do exercises aimed at strengthening one set of muscles on one day and then switch to another set of muscles on the second day—quadriceps and ankles one day and arm muscles another day.

The super-slows. This group argues that exercising at a snail's pace increases results. A Texas physician, who claimed he once ran sixty miles a week, is now exercising only twenty minutes a week, using the super-slow format. He claims he gets the same amount of exercise benefit out of his twenty minutes of super-slow exercising as he got when he ran those sixty miles every week. He does ten repetitions for each exercise with each rep taking fourteen seconds.

The Texas doctor's pace is really too slow for us unsteady Seniors, as you will find if you try it. Don provides guidelines for different types of exercise in his chapters. Some of us, when we exercise, have a tendency to speed and bounce along through our exercises as if to get them over as soon as possible. As Don will suggest, slowing down a little is not a bad idea. As we age, speed is a recipe for injury.

Interval training. Some exercise researchers have discovered that fast and then slow adds to the benefits of exercise for cardiovascular fitness.

One trainer suggests a warm up walk of two minutes, then fifteen seconds at a faster speed, and then a minute at regular speed. Then fifteen seconds, etc., for six repetitions. It will increase endurance over a short period of weeks. We can use this in walking, cycling, or swimming.

But interval training is definitely not for those with heart disease or high blood pressure. Unsteady Seniors, check with your physician first.

Sets for Seniors. One expert recommends that Seniors do only one set of strengthening exercises for twelve repetitions but to the maximum weight you can handle. This will accomplish the same result, he says, as three sets at lower weights. His theory has yet to be proven. Don will recommend the generally accepted procedure for each type of exercise.

Correct-posture exercises. We could call these the Leaning Tower of Pisa exercises. We know if a building isn't perpendicular to the ground, it will eventually fall down from its own weight (unless buttressed or using steel beams). Gravity is the villain that makes that Pisa tower lean.

Those who emphasize correct posture argue that our bodies should be as close to perpendicular to the ground as possible—what they call vertical alignment. Without vertical alignment, they claim we Seniors will have trouble with balance because we are tilted.

Callantics. This technique builds correct posture through a variety of techniques with overlaps to Pilates core training, ballet, Tai Chi, and even Yoga, but they put the primary emphasis squarely and on getting used to having correct posture.

The Alexander Technique. Frederick Alexander invented a technique that is similar. It also stresses the correct alignment of the head, neck, and spine. The instructor tells you what's wrong and makes corrections with a series of gentle touches.

Correct-posture techniques. We all remember how ladies in finishing schools used to train themselves to a stately posture by walking around with books balanced on their heads. A variation for today is called the Level-Headed Hat. The hat gives a nasty signal if you dare to slouch.

Other suggestions are that we unsteady Seniors wear a striped shirt—it shows misalignments. Imagine the crown of our head reaching up to the ceiling or just keeping a mirror handy by our easy chairs to check ourselves.

Stretching exercises. My doctor friend tells me that the elasticity in our muscles begins declining at—guess what age. At thirty, he says! And particularly so as we glide pass sixty-five, and especially so for those of us Seniors who have been sedentary. So for us, a little stretching will increase, or help us regain, our range of motion and flexibility and should be part of our exercise routine.

Two major studies were begun in 2007 to determine the effects of stretching, especially whether stretching will prevent soreness and possible injuries. Studies are being done jointly in Norway and Australia and the other in the United States by USA Track & Field.

Whether stretching exercises prevent injuries has been challenged in a number of smaller studies. Coaches and trainers vary in their use. Some favor stretching before exercising, others after, and some never. Don reflects on this problem and then recommends certain flexibility exercises for us unsteady Seniors while he advises against others.

Resistance stretching. This form of stretching was used by Dara Torres who, at forty-one, swam in the 2008 summer Olympics in China, the oldest person to ever compete. She won three silver medals. The exercise requires flexing your muscles as you stretch—an eccentric contraction.

Thus, on a leg lift, you don't relax your muscles but gradually lower the weight as the muscle lengthens.

WHAT ALL THESE RESEARCHES MEAN FOR US UNSTEADY SENIORS

Most of these researches are still in the clinical trial stage. Knowing help is on the way should give us hope. And some of these discoveries are already helping unsteady Seniors.

THE HOPEFUL RESEARCH GOING ON
WHAT WAS THAT CHAPTER ALL ABOUT?

The cutting-edge research on balance is on how to reactivate the sensors at the bottom of our feet and the nerves that make up our communication system. Researchers are also studying how to reeducate our brains to regain position sense. And practitioners are designing exercises aimed at specific problems.

Chapter 3

THE UNSTEADY SENIOR REVIEWS
PRACTITIONER TREATMENTS

Some of the therapies proposed by practitioners do not fit neatly into any of the research categories. A number are based on a theory, or perhaps we should call it an unproven hypothesis. From it, the practitioners derive techniques they suggest will help cure our balance difficulties. Sometimes a technique works for some and not for others. Just because it is inspired, its effectiveness must still be validated.

Some are included in this handbook since I think we unsteady Seniors should be aware of all that's out there that might help us. A few of the techniques described here are widely used while others are hardly known. One of the latter is my first entry.

Isometric twitching. Semyon Krewer, an atomic physicist, had severe but not completely crippling arthritis. He and physical therapist Ann Edgar developed over three hundred exercises for a program for arthritics requiring five minutes of exercise in the morning and five to fifteen minutes each evening to increase muscle strength and range of motion. The morning exercises were a circuit of twenty-three exercises of tense-relax-and-stretch routines. Each evening session throughout the week was designed to exercise a different part of the body.

Krewer also taught himself to do a unique isometric exercise—exercises that strengthen muscles without actually moving painful joints. Once a day, he contracted (twitched) a muscle as strongly as possible for three to six seconds. This twitching, he claimed, extends over the period of six weeks to achieve the maximum strength possible for that muscle.

But Krewer also found twitches useful for relaxation. He did a slow muscle twitch from one to three seconds.

And he also recommended short, fast, and forceful twitches of one second each for up to twenty times. They are useful for building endurance and rebuilding strength.

Through these contractions, he says that he taught himself to simulate the muscles used in biking and jogging without moving his painful joints or getting out of his chair. After a period of illness requiring prolonged bed rest, he found he was unable to raise himself on his toes or lift his left arm. For two days, he did up to fifty fast-twitching exercises throughout the day. He was then able to raise his toes five to ten times and lift two pound weights with his left arm.

Krewer notes it took him a while to learn to do his exercise twitches for the quads and hamstrings. Take it for what it's worth.

His book is Semyon Krewer and Ann Edgar's *The Arthritis Exercise Book, A Comprehensive Program for Controlling the Effects of Arthritis While Relieving Pain*, NY: Simon & Schuster, 1981.

Muscle Activation Techniques (MAT). Greg Roskpf is a Denver-based exercise physiologist and biomechanical consultant for the Denver Broncos, the Denver Nuggets, and the Utah Jazz. When he was nineteen, he fractured a vertebra which led to back, hip, and knee pain. He tried various treatments but none helped very much.

His focus then shifted from pain control to muscle physiology. His theory is that the sensitizers of some muscles stopped sending messages from the brain to a muscle, and the muscle then became weak from disuse. Next, the opposing muscle tightened up to reduce the range of motion in order to protect the weak nonfunctioning muscle.

He assesses a person's range of motion from neck to toe. Next, the related nonfunctioning muscles are checked to determine if they contract when messages are sent from the brain. If not, strong pressure back and forth in an *X* pattern is applied to where those muscles grow into the bones. This is where he believes the lazy sensitizers are located. After being stimulated, the sensitizers should once again receive messages from the brain. Finally, the muscles are rechecked to see whether range of motion and strength is restored.

Bonnie Keth in an article for the *Chicago Tribune* of August 13, 2005 described the case of a woman who lost the motion of her thumb. Surgeons recommended an operation. She regained motion when the MAT therapist applied pressure to points at her neck and shoulders.

Yoga. This was developed five thousand years ago in India. Besides physical fitness, it offers, and I quote from a local advertisement, "an open and cleansed mind, body, and spirit." Yoga emphasizes reducing stress but also promises many physical benefits, and again I quote, "increase range of motion, relaxes the muscles, builds strength, aids in skeletal and muscle alignment, relieves pain, keeps you feeling younger, and increases blood flow—bringing blood into areas of the body that have great long-term rewarding benefits."

Yoga incorporates deep and free breathing through the nose and stopping to focus your mind during the rests between movements. Yoga emphasizes precision and proper alignment of body parts, expanding the range of motion for every joint, with slow movements, and holding a pose (asanas). Yoga uses body weight to provide the resistance that strengthens the muscles and increases range of motion. Each exercise stops after three repetitions.

A number of Yoga variations exist. Hatha is designed for beginners. Lyengar emphasizes precise alignment along with strength.

Restorative yoga emphasizes relaxation. Other practices are designed to work up a sweat, raise your heart rate, or sculpt the body.

Some of the body position poses may well be difficult for us unsteady Seniors. Others seem to have wandered out of Yoga into our balance exercise programs without crediting their Yoga origins.

We unsteady Seniors are advised to begin with the simple poses. In one article, a Yoga teacher is quoted as starting Seniors by lying on their backs and "stretching one leg straight up with a strap over the sole of the foot," a standard balance exercise. An alternative Yoga for Seniors is called chair yoga. This set of positions was developed especially for those who can't do some of the regular poses.

Massage. The major claim for massage is that it provides deep relaxation, and that alone should make it attractive for us unsteady Seniors. Massage will also loosen tight muscles aiding in flexibility.

A good massage therapist can release knotted muscles. If we have a strain, they can ease our pain.

For more information, look up the website of the American Massage Therapy Association at www.amtamassage.org.

Myofascial release massage. Below the skin and covering the muscles is a layer of something called the fascia. My doctor friend described the fascia as a thin membrane that covers the whole body.

When we are injured, the fascia, massagers claim, gets stuck to and tangled with a nearby muscle. The prescribed massage is a series of skin rolls to loosen the fascia layer and separate it from the muscle.

ART (Active Release Technique). Dr. P. Michael Leahy, a former aerospace engineer, became a doctor of chiropractic, developed and patented ART in 1988 as a system for treating pain, stiffness, tendinitis, and loss of range of motion caused by soft tissue injury. Some eight NFL teams now use ART.

The theory is that overuse of muscles, or an injury, may result in scar tissue and adhesions, which may lead to small tears, inflammation, and restricted movement. The scar tissue buildup prevents the soft tissue from moving normally. Soft tissue includes the fascia, ligaments, muscles, tendons, and nerves.

The treatment consists of diagnosis followed by one or more of the five hundred specific "moves" the therapist can choose, each aimed at a specific soft tissue condition. The ART practitioner finds the scar tissue and applies pressure with the thumb. At the same time, the patient shortens and then elongates the muscle to a fully stretched position.

Rolfing, also known as structural integration. Ida P. Rolf, PhD, who invented Rolfing, was born in 1896. She earned a doctorate in biological chemistry from Columbia University in 1920 and then worked at the Rockefeller Institute. She invented Rolfing to deal with family health problems. At age seventy-six, she established the Rolf Institute of Structural Integration located in Boulder, Colorado.

Rolfing assumes the fascia, the layer that covers the muscles, becomes shorter and tightens, and this pulls the body out of proper alignment. Knocks and bad habits are thought to have pushed or pulled these out of line. The practitioner manipulates the body's connective tissue and stretches its muscles to restore proper alignment.

To accomplish better alignment, a Rolfer either hits or applies pressure with the fingertips, forearm, or elbow to free up adhesions that are constricting muscles, joints, and bones. The technique sometimes requires ten sessions of from sixty to ninety minutes.

Is this painful? Yes, sometimes, so those who have gone through Rolfing report. But the converted say it works and is scientific and is worth the pain and cost.

Acupuncture. Here's another Chinese import. Most of us think of acupuncture as its name suggests—poking needles about the thickness of a human hair under the skin into nerves at approximately 365 specified points. They then stay in place from five minutes to half an hour.

They are said to send messages to the brain to release soothing hormones. The treatments last from several days to several weeks and are relatively painless. Treatments may also be done with finger, hand, and arm pressure, electric currents, magnets, and a half a dozen other methods, including, for the way out, bee stings.

The theory behind all this is that an energy force called qi (chee) flows through the body along channels called meridians—twelve primary and eight secondary ones. This energy is of competing forces: yin (cold and sluggish) and its opposite, yang (hot and animated). A blockage in these channels causes disease and pain. Stimulating the meridians at certain points breaks up the blockages and makes us more able to control our movements.

So far, researchers have been unable to locate any of these meridians, though they note that many of the acupuncture stimulus points are places where we find nerve endings.

In 1996, the Food and Drug Administration approved needles for licensed practitioners. The needles muse be sterile and only used once.

All but eight states also now certify acupuncture practitioners. Some health plans cover the cost of acupuncture.

Acupuncture seems to work especially well for some conditions such as nausea, migraines, asthma, lower back pain, and perhaps the stiffness of arthritis. But it seems to work selectively. Some patients are helped, but others are not.

The National Institutes of Health evaluated the effectiveness of acupuncture. Some experiments used acupuncture and what they called sham acupuncture (the needles placed at random). They found the same level of improvement from both. This suggested to some the placebo effect, that because patients expected to improve, they did.

Other researchers suggested that the brain was reacting to punctures wherever they occurred. These skeptics suggested the needles caused the central nervous system to release pain killers called endorphins.

But an important finding was that brain scans revealed that acupuncture stimulated some parts of the brain and suppressed others.

The over 14,000 American acupuncturists includes three thousand doctors and some dentists. To check on credentials of your neighborhood acupuncturist, contact the Accreditation Commission for Acupuncture and Oriental Medicine at www.acaom.org or for physicians who do acupuncture: the American Academy of Medical Acupuncture in Los Angeles at www.medicalacupuncture.org. Also, about one-third of the members of the American Massage Therapy Association offer acupressure. Check at www.amtamassage.org.

Reflexology. This is a kind of near relation to acupuncture, though its practitioners claim it dates from 2300 BC and was developed in Iraq. The theory is that crystalline deposits of uric acid form at some 7,200 nerve endings restricting circulation.

By breaking up the deposits, circulation is restored, the body is relaxed, and the process thereby stimulates the body's own healing process. The professional puts pressure through the hands and fingers at certain places on our hands or at the bottom of our feet where they say 7,200 nerve endings flourish.

As in acupuncture, each pressure point is theorized to affect a different part of our body, often far distant from the pressure point. Machines are now available that cause weak electric shocks on these pressure points but individuals with pacemakers are warned not to use them.

Chiropractic. The basic theory here is that the body has "an innate intelligence" to bring about cures, unless the vertebrae get out of alignment. Such a condition interferes with communication throughout the nervous system which prevents the body from functioning properly. The treatment is called spinal adjustment.

Chiropractors have also been especially successful in adjusting other body parts. Many injured athletes have found chiropractic helpful in relieving pain and stiffness. And some use it just to feel good.

The Feldenkrais Method. This one only dates back to half a century ago. A Russian-born physicist Moshe Feldendkrais argued that we all moved correctly as children, but as some of us age, we drift away from proper movements. So we have to reeducate our bodies. Proper movement is regained by the practitioner telling you what you are doing wrong and using gentle touch to make corrections.

Cobblestone walking. Many parks in China have cobblestone walks. The Chinese claim that walking on them helps the balance problems of unsteady Seniors as well as strengthening leg muscles.

Researchers in Oregon checked this out with special mats and found it had some validity. But they advise that we unsteady Seniors shouldn't go trying this at home on our own.

Walking in Sand. This looks like a variation of cobblestone walking and also is a more practical, particularly if you fall. The researchers tell us unsteady Seniors who are ploughing along through loose sand are boosting our energy expenditures by a third. Don suggests which unsteady Seniors should avoid those beach walks.

The trouble is that when I walk the beach, I tend to go close to the shore where the sand is wet and hard and easier to walk on rather than, as I should, struggle along in the hot sun in drier sand.

Actually, if the sand is level and not slanted, walking on wet sand is among the best surfaces for those with weak knees. It is not hard like concrete sidewalks or blacktop roads or as difficult as walking in loose sand. It has just the right amount of give.

PRACTITIONER TREATMENTS
WHAT WAS THAT CHAPTER ALL ABOUT?

A number of other therapies also hold out some promise for help to relieve balance difficulties, and more of these are now facing experimental testing. For some of these treatments, the theory may be unproven but the technique still may work, though not always for every person.

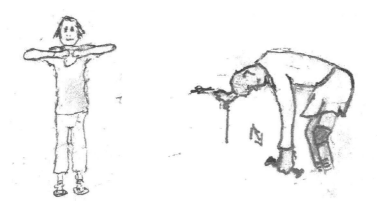

Chapter 4

The Unsteady Senior Asks

Who Is Most Likely to Fall?

Even athletic twenty-year-olds lose their balance and fall and maybe even break an arm or leg. But they don't seem to engage in these kind of acrobatics as often as we unsteady Seniors do or have as serious results when they do.

We all know that the chances that we may fall increase as we get older. Those over sixty-five fall at least once a year on average, or so we unsteady Seniors are told.

So before going further, let's take a look at who among us is the unsteady Senior most likely to fall.

What Researchers Say About Chances of a Serious Fall

Dr. Mary Tinetti is director of the Yale Program on Aging. She heads a major unit doing research on balance among Seniors.

She claims that the major reasons for our balance problems are the diminished senses of touch and position (proprioception) and adds a new factor—our reflexes slow as we age.

Serious falls, Dr. Tinetti and her associates found, are more than just bad luck. Some Seniors are more likely to have such falls. She and her associates limited their study of those who had suffered falls that caused a hip fracture.

Falls in the home. Researchers found that about 75 percent of falls occur in the home. Despite what this might suggest, they didn't find that hazards in the home were a major cause of serious falls. This doesn't mean that commonsense precautions shouldn't be followed. Dr. Tinetti is hell on wheels for getting rid of throw rugs.

It is possible though that many unsteady Seniors have already corrected the obvious hazards. But if you want to check for yourself, you can review Chapter 12, "Hazards around the Home."

The reason for the 75 percent finding is that Seniors spend a lot more time in their homes after they retire. So home is where the other conditions that raise the chances of a serious fall will occur.

Those most at risk of a serious fall. Note how many of the victims that Dr. Tinetti identified as likely to be vulnerable are already weakened in one way or another, generally by disease.

1. *Arthritis.* Arthritic Seniors become stiff and movement becomes painful. Range of motion gets more restricted and movements are less under their control.

2. *Impaired vision.* This includes reduced vision, blindness, the presence of cataracts, wearing out-of-date prescription glasses, or not getting glasses when you need them. It even includes such acts as wearing reading glasses when walking about or keeping on sun glasses at twilight or after dark. Glasses that get fogged also may cause a fall. Bifocals may give Seniors trouble with depth perception when looking down, especially so on stairs. Some experts say get one pair for reading and another for distance.

Note that Dr. Tinetti uses the words "impaired vision" to describe anything that blocks our ability to see where we're going (includes dim lighting or glare). Our eyes are the major aid we unsteady Seniors have in navigating.

3. *Loss of muscle strength.* The very frail are most in danger of a serious fall, but that doesn't let off the rest of us couch potatoes. Weak muscles increase the dangers for all of us unsteady Seniors.

4. *Dementia.*

5. *Taking four or more prescription medicines*. This includes especially anti-depressants, epilepsy, and heart medications. A mix of medicines that different specialists recommend, each for a different problem, may interact and cause dizziness.
6. *Osteoporosis*. Bone thinning.
7. *Light-headedness*.

OTHER CAUSES

A recent study at the University of Michigan suggests that unsteady Seniors can add another reason that people fall.

Insomnia. Doctors used to hesitate to prescribe sleeping pills to us Seniors for fear that the medication would continue to confuse us after we wake up. But newer pills leave our system faster, and so we can be better at limiting the impact of the pills to when we sleep.

Doctors at the University of Michigan made a study of thirty-four thousand nursing home residents over a six month period. Those with untreated insomnia were 90 percent more likely to fall than other residents.

Those insomniacs given sleeping pills were only 29 percent more likely to fall. We all know why. Whenever we go without sleep, our reaction times are slower, and we are less mentally alert.

Muscle performance is also affected but in a way that may surprise the unsteady Senior. Those who went without sleep, thought they were more capable of getting around than they really were, could lead to falls as well, parenthetically, to auto accidents.

Dr. Alon Avidan, who supervised the study, said the researchers received no funds from the pharmaceutical industry—a nice touch, I thought.

Medications that affect alertness. Sleeping pills can be risky for unsteady Seniors, but there are others as well. Dr. John Morley of Washington University says that other medications that affect alertness are antidepressants, antipsychotics, antianxiety drugs, and antihistamines.

Some studies also have found a higher risk of falling among Seniors who take diuretics, which help lower blood pressure.

When researchers in the Netherlands cut the overuse of these "fall-risk-increasing drugs" for seventy-five people, for all sixty-five and over, the number of falls was cut in half.

Vitamin D deficiency. *D* is the sunshine vitamin. Those of us Seniors, like Don and me, who live in northern climates like Michigan, where the clouds roll in off the Big Lake starting in fall, get less sunlight all winter and are advised to take vitamin D pills.

A year-long study of 1231 adults over sixty-five (Consumer Reports—November 2006), found that individuals deficient in vitamin D were 78 percent more likely to fall than those with adequate vitamin D levels.

Diabetes. Researchers at Columbia University studied 139 residents of a home for the aged ranging in age from 70 to 105. They found that, within a period of almost three hundred days, four out of five residents with diabetes, including those with Type 2 diabetes, had a fall (80 percent), as compared to one in three (33 percent) of residents without diabetes. Complications of diabetes may include vision problems as well as peripheral nerve damage.

Protein deficiency. Lack of protein has been found to cause muscles to atrophy and become weaker and is thus less likely to prevent a fall. Dr. Wayne Campbell, a professor of Foods and Nutrition at Purdue University, found 25 percent of two thousand men and women aged sixty-five to eighty-five were consuming inadequate amounts of protein. Researchers found the desire to eat higher protein foods was reduced, especially in Seniors living alone. Their diets often became heavier with more carbohydrates, such as toast and jam.

WHAT THE STUDIES TELL US UNSTEADY SENIORS

When we unsteady Seniors look over this list of what leads to serious falls, we first of all note some causes of falls that don't apply to most of us—dementia, blindness, being very frail, and being diabetic.

We also see diabetes as being more important than age in causing falls. Serious falls most often hit the walking wounded. But unfortunately most of the diseases listed here are those that commonly afflict Seniors, and some perhaps go undiagnosed.

Medications. Medical specialists tend to treat their disease specialty, sometimes without considering the effect on what other specialists prescribe. Thus we can have a mixture of medications that lead to problems of balance. Even some vitamins may disturb the mix.

Some necessary medications such as diuretics or antidepressants or over-the-counter drugs such as antihistamines or sleeping pills result in our being less alert that can also lead to serious falls.

Checking with your doctor. The first thing I did back when I got serious about this balance thing was to have my family doctor check me out. She had my medical records and knew my medical history and was able to make useful suggestions.

My doctor also said a few words about arthritis and its treatment. Way before knee operations, I knew the NSAID that worked for me.

She sent me to a neurologist. He diagnosed peripheral neuropathy, though I was neither a diabetic nor an alcoholic. The nerves about six inches down from my knees had given up trying to get accurate balance signals from the important sensors at the bottom of my feet and had sometimes garbled information to send up to mission central.

There are three types of nerves: Sensory nerves transmit sensations like hot or cold or and when stubbing your toe—pain. Autonomic nerves regulate functions that are not under conscious control like blood pressure. The problem I have is with the motor nerves, which control the actions of muscles throughout the body and so affect balance.

After a time, I've concluded that perhaps many other unsteady Seniors have undiagnosed peripheral neuropathy of the motor type. That's what the researchers at the cutting edge seem to think with all the emphasis on the sensors on the soles of our feet.

Recently an ad in the *Chicago Tribune* suggested that I might not be wrong about this. It was promoting a therapy for people with peripheral neuropathy "including those nondiabetics with neuropathy symptoms." The ad listed five treatment centers that had already sprung up around the Chicago suburbs, which suggests someone out there thinks a great many of us unsteady Seniors, with money to spend, are in need of their services.

Since I have a lazy eye, I also have regularly had my eyes checked regularly since about age five.

FINDING AND TREATING OUR INDIVIDUAL PROBLEMS

Many unsteady Seniors have arthritis, some osteoporosis, and others diabetes. It's good to remember that we Seniors do not all have the same physical problems that affect our unsteadiness. Also, recognize that our known deficiencies may change overtime.

Dr. Tinetti points to the advice given doctors—treat the patient rather than the disease. One prescription doesn't fit all.

FOR STARTERS 1

Check in with your physician to correct, to the extent possible, any debilitating conditions and have him or her review the medications, drugs, and vitamins you are taking.

INDIVIDUAL TREATMENTS

The head trainer of the Chicago White Sox, Herm Schneider, has some excellent advice for us unsteady Seniors. The Championship White Sox of 2005 won in part because the team had an exercise program designed to keep players off the disabled list. This program was tailored to the needs of individual players.

Pitchers had a different set of exercises than center fielders; those exercises even varied on the days before and after they pitched. Exercises done between seasons were different from those after the season began.

We begin with our own individual problems and, as Don will suggest, tailor our exercise program to our own individual problems.

FOR STARTERS 2

Expect Don's chapters to systematically begin with a series of tests of your own posture, balance, and muscle strength to determine your individual weaknesses.

However, balance is our common problem, and we all can benefit from balance, flexibility, and strengthening exercises.

FOR STARTERS 3

Expect Don to recommend exercises for balance, flexibility, and strengthening tailored for unsteady Seniors.

But before that happens, we have some distance to travel, starting with taking a look at what really keeps us from getting started and useful suggestions on other matters.

Expect more "FOR STARTERS."

WHO IS MOST LIKELY TO FALL?
WHAT WAS THAT CHAPTER ALL ABOUT?

Those Seniors most in danger of serious falls are the walking wounded—weakened most often by disease, not including age. So a first step before handling your unsteadiness is to check in with your physician.

Each Senior has individual weaknesses contributing to unsteadiness that require specific exercises. But all of us also have a common problem of unsteadiness, and we will benefit from a general set of balance, flexibility, and strengthening exercises.

Don's chapters will help you tailor an exercise program that addresses both of these conditions.

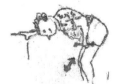

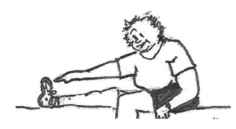

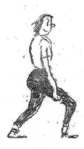

Chapter 5

The Unsteady Senior Asks

So What Prevents Us from Getting Started?

We Seniors all recognize that research always promise that breakthroughs are coming. But they always seem to be about five years away, and that's a little longer time than it used to be, after we speed past age sixty-five.

So we need to make a start right now with what the researchers have found out.

What we all desire. Lady Mary Wortley Montagu spelled it out—what it is that we unsteady Seniors all want for ourselves.

"To die young, BUT, as late as possible."

None of us unsteady Seniors is quite ready to be put on the shelf. We want to stay independent, celebrate a pleasant and fulfilling life as long as we're around—to stay active—live and enjoy.

What the medical experts tell us. The key to staying young, the medical experts proclaim over and over, is: *stay active!*

They are even pretty blunt about this. They say we Seniors have no choice: to stay active or to get ready to die.

The medical researchers promise us a satisfying life if we stay active. They say that loss of balance is not inevitable as we get older. They say that we can improve our balance if we work at it.

They have found that every little bit of activity pays off for us. A Harvard group who studied sixty-one thousand Senior women over a twelve-year period found that those who got up out of their chairs and just stood up, just for ten hours a week, reduced the risk of hip fractures by 28 percent. If we consider the group who stood for fifty-five hours a week or more, the reduction was 46 percent. That's just standing, nothing more (unless one or two of those women actually took a step or two and didn't report it to the researchers). Just kidding!

Researchers have found that activity even stirs up our genes. Bernadine Healy, the MD who did the "On Health" column in *U.S. News and World Report,* wrote in the June 16, 2006 issue, "More than 140 exercise-related genes are awakened if the body gets off the couch and engages in physical activity. These sleeping beauties make proteins with wide ranging benefits to . . ." We Seniors get the point.

So What Stands in the Way of Our Getting Active?

The process, in part, it's not knowing what we can do to improve our strength and balance. Don will sort that out later on in his chapters. But it may really be something else.

A basic fear for many unsteady Seniors is that they might fall and break some of their precious physical equipment. We sometimes hear it when Seniors get together to talk about being a little unsteady.

"If I fall, my kids will put me into a nursing home."

The fear of falling. According to the researchers, some unsteady Seniors begin to let just the fear of falling restrict their activity—between 30 to 50 percent get that way according to one estimate made after polling Seniors in a residence home.

We Seniors know that the only sure way to avoid falling is rarely to get out of bed or easy chairs and if we do, to hang on to something or somebody. If we really want to be absolutely safe, we could crawl around on the floor to get where we want to go. That's a ridiculous caricature of the way some Seniors live but not too far off.

I'm reminded of a Lonesome George Gobel joke about how on New Year's eve he had a little too much of liquid stimulators. He started home and almost made it, and then some clown stepped on his hand. We Seniors don't want that to happen to us.

The Worst Thing We Unsteady Seniors Can Do

Because of the fear of falling, some unsteady Seniors sharply restrict their activities, beginning even with such basic acts as standing up and walking. Something like a whirlpool of potential calamity begins slowly swirling around them. They get overly cautious, more sedentary, steadily weaker, more and more unsteady and weaker still, and then one day get drawn down into the maelstrom of a serious fall.

So the dread of potential calamity becomes a self-fulfilling prophecy. This does not make for a very happy present or a pleasant future to look forward to either.

Every activity has *some risk*, but allowing yourself to become inactive has even *more risk*.

Irrational fears. We unsteady Seniors get reminded, too often perhaps, of what one of our greatest presidents said about fear at a critical moment in our nation's history.

"So, first of all, let me assert my firm belief that the only thing we have to fear is fear itself."

But FDR didn't stop there as some people who like to quote him do. He wasn't saying that all fears are imaginary. He went on to describe precisely the kind of fears he was warning against: "nameless, unreasonable, unjustified terror which paralyzes needed efforts to convert retreat into advance."

Hysterical terrors that paralyze us, fears which have no basis in reality—these are the kind of fears President Roosevelt was warning against. These hold too many unsteady Seniors in chains and shackles.

We unsteady Seniors have to somehow face down these imaginary and irrational fears if we are to improve. It's a *must* because it's the only way we will improve. Unless we stay reasonably active, we can forget about a more normal life.

Overcoming imaginary fears about falling may not be easy for some. What can we say to them? Some will shout that they can't be cowards, build up your courage; to be brave, act brave; etc.

But let's just settle for something a little less daunting, just be *willing to try.* If we unsteady Seniors are willing to try, there's hope.

Dr Steve Blair, an epidemiologist at the University of South Carolina whose research formed much of the basis for the federal exercise guidelines says, "A one minute walk isn't going to do much for your health, but it is a way to start. Next week, can you do two minutes? Advance to three minutes the third week. Eventually, you'll be up to 30." And he points out it doesn't have to be done all at once. You can do ten minutes in the morning and ten in the afternoon.

The important thing is to begin and a willingness to try.

When unsteady Seniors begin to face down irrational fears by being willing to try those first steps, they choose the path back to a more active life. We unsteady Seniors then start on the journey that ends in opening the door to what will really help with our unsteadiness.

FOR STARTERS 4

On our own, we have to be willing to try to become more active and thereby overcome our irrational fears and take the first big and basic step toward recovery. We have to decide by ourselves. No one else can do it for us.

Rational Fears

President Franklin Roosevelt was a polio victim who could only maneuver with a cane and holding on to someone. Most of the time, he got around in a wheel chair. He had taken his share of knocks and falls. He knew that concrete sidewalks weren't made of marshmallows.

FDR knew of threats out there that weren't *nameless*—we unsteady Seniors have little trouble identifying what hurrying down a steep staircase might do for us. And he could name other fears as well that weren't *unreasonable* or *unjustified*.

Roosevelt's greatest fear was of fire, a reasonable and justified one for him. After he realized he would be handicapped for some time to come, he began practicing how to escape in case of fire. He began painfully pulling himself across the floor and crawling out his bedroom along a prearranged route to safety.

While in the White House, he retired the presidential yacht *Sequoia*" that President Hoover had used because it had a wooden hull that could go up in flames. FDR's presidential yacht, *The Potomac*," had a steel hull. That is recognizing justified fears and doing something about them.

The real dangers. What are the real risks we unsteady Seniors face? If we think about it, we begin to realize that it isn't taking the big risks. Most of us don't climb on roofs anymore. A roof is for those under forty.

The last time I was on a roof, I almost got trapped up there. When the time came to get down, I stood up there thinking long thoughts. I had to swing my unsteady leg out over open space in order to put it on the top rung of that ladder. Nance never heard about this, until later. Roof dancing, I decided then, is for Santa's reindeers.

Most of us also probably steer clear of skydiving-jumping out of planes with just a flimsy parachute that might not open, as one of our Senior ex-presidents does from time to time as a hobby.

What are the foolish risks? The real hazards for us are doing things we used to do so casually back in the past without thinking about it. Now they have become silly little chances we are tempted to take and still feel we can get away with. Those are the real risks.

We want to get that bottle of ketchup on the top shelf, and we want it right now, and no one else is around to help. We climb up on a chair so we can reach far out for that precious bottle of red goo.

Or we forgot something and go back into a darkened room, in too much of a hurry to stop and turn on the light switch. Or we want the morning paper to read with our morning coffee, and so we go sailing out on to a snow-covered driveway to snag it before our coffee gets cold.

It's these smaller and more commonplace activities that tempt us to take foolish risks. And those are the risks that spell trouble.

Guides for deciding. We know we must face down irrational doubts and fears. We have to start out being willing to try. But we also know some dangers are real. So the problem boils down to finding a balance between the trying and not taking foolish risks.

The first rule is *not to be impatient*, which for me is easier said than done. Impatience often fuels the foolishness that causes us to risk a spill. Impatience is inevitably the enemy for unsteady Seniors,

Next, we have to try to be *realistic about our own strength and unsteadiness*, knowing what we can do and what we probably can't do. It's that old listen to what your body is telling you thing. Otherwise we will have to learn the hard way through trial and error.

We have to use *commonsense prudence*, what the Oxford dictionary defines as "showing care and forethought."

Those two phrases can solve a lot of problems for us, so I'll capitalize them: SHOWING CARE and FORETHOUGHT.

Showing care. Occasionally, we need to stop for a second and take a second look. There's an old saying, "Look before you leap," and if we don't stop to look, limping around is what we may have to do. It's like that old carpentry advice—measure twice, saw once.

Forethought. That is the reason to keep a cane in the car or to take one to the movies, even though you may not need it. It is also the reason for getting rid of throw rugs and putting in hand grips and having unimpeded stairs, subjects we cover in a later chapter.

And some risks are too great even if the odds of succeeding are pretty good. Like playing Russian roulette with loaded pistols (five to one odds), the result, if we lose though, isn't nice.

Have I always followed these guidelines?

Read on, Oh Unsteady Seniors, read on.

MEMORABLE FALLS I HAVE PERSONALLY PARTICIPATED IN

Like most of us Seniors, I often think that I'm about fifteen years younger than I really am, which is perhaps why I haven't always been prudent and used good common sense. But another side of me remembers what the ageless pitcher Satchel Paige came up with, "How old would you be if you didn't know how old you was?"

Let me illustrate using some of my own sad experiences in this school of hard knocks.

The first fall I recall vividly might happen to anyone. Still it's an especially hazardous activity for unsteady Seniors—going down the basement stairs carrying a big box. I couldn't see my feet or hold on to the rail. I thought I was at the bottom. I only missed the step count by one.

So I blissfully stepped out into airy space and then sprawled onto the floor, which fortunately was carpeted. All I did was skin an ankle, but my head just missed the corner of a bookcase. As we unsteady Seniors know, the most serious injuries from falls are hip fractures and injuries to the head. The other most common injuries are to the forearm or wrists. I was lucky.

At our cottage, I once walked out the door and was taking the one step down to the ground while at the same time using the remote to open the trunk of the car when—boom! I miss stepped. The lesson I suppose is that we shouldn't try to do two things at once, especially when we're moving down steps. President Lyndon Johnson said of one of his opponents that he couldn't walk and chew gum at the same time, and I guess I'm almost there sometimes too.

And then, another time, I walked into a darkened room to get something and got tangled up in the wires from my desktop computer. It was so stupid; I don't even want to talk about it.

But I've saved the best to last. If I could just remember how I did it, I could patent it and sell it to every physical therapy clinic.

We were unloading the stuff that we brought home from the cottage at the end of the summer into the basement freezer. Then I started back upstairs dragging the cooler behind me, still full of those frozen blue blocks. When I got to the top step, I let go of the railing to pull me and the ice box up over the top and—*wham!* The cooler pulled me back. Of the twelve steps, I figure I only missed the top three. Again, I was lucky—just cuts and bruises.

I didn't give a thought about the weight of a cooler full of blue ice blocks and so overestimated my own strength.

As Don will later tell you on how to fall, no one can teach you how to fall down a flight of stairs without hurting yourself. All I can tell you if you want to try it is—be lucky! If you have to fall, try a short fall forward going up and a quick fall back on your fanny going down.

I can't be sure about this, but maybe my not getting hurt suggests that all that exercising pays off in some unexpected ways.

One thing I've noticed about my falls is that nearly always no one else has been around to see me take the tumble. This I can't explain. Maybe I'm more impatient or devil-may-care when no one else is around to shout, "Charlie, don't do that!" Or I forget I'm not as young as I used to be, and I take those unnecessary risks. I don't know why for sure. I just know it is.

MY FALLS HAVE ALL BEEN MY OWN FAULT

You may think this is not a very comforting thought, until you think about it. It means the falls I've taken were not my inevitable lot as an unsteady Senior. My falls were falls that could have been prevented. I can't remember anyone else ever knocking me down.

This means we unsteady Seniors can live an active life while having it in our power to drastically reduce the probability we will fall.

A FUTURE WITHOUT FALLS?

Will we be prudent and use commonsense to ensure we will never fall again? We all wish it were so, but no one can guarantee that.

We are all sinners and backsliders and not always as sensible as we should be. We make mistakes about our own strength or ability or fail to see the dangers ahead, or we are just sometimes ornery enough to take unnecessary chances even when we know we shouldn't.

And the world out there is full of blood, toil, tears, and sweat, as someone observed. With our age and our balance problems, we know we are at a disadvantage, and, at some time, the luck may break against us. We may be run down by a gang of unruly kids on skateboards.

By using common sense and prudence (showing care and forethought), knowing our own strength and not being impatient, we are taking the first step toward sharply reducing the probabilities of a fall. It's the probabilities that are important for us unsteady Seniors.

FOR STARTERS 5

Be willing to try to be active, but be prudent using common sense care and forethought, and don't be so impatient.

CALCULATED RISKS

But that's not the whole story. There are calculated risks. As a paraplegic, Franklin Roosevelt knew he would be helpless in a fiery airplane crash. Yet only five years after Lindbergh flew the Atlantic, when flying was still a risky novelty, FDR had himself flown, bucking storms and strong headwinds, requiring several takeoffs and landings to refuel.

FDR wanted to accept the presidential nomination in person at the Democratic National Convention of 1932. Until then, nominees waited around for a month or so until party leaders got around to calling to inform them, in case they hadn't noticed, that a major party had nominated them for president.

He decided the nation in the depths of the Great Depression needed an electrifying example of a new leadership—a new deal. So he gritted his teeth and took a calculated risk. But he didn't fly again for ten years, not until he soared off to meet Churchill and Stalin during World War II—another calculated risk. But, even then, he was known to talk to others about his fear of fire if the plane crashed.

Emergencies may force us unsteady Seniors very, very infrequently to take calculated risks. Some saved in Katrina's disastrous floods in New Orleans were unsteady Seniors who had to climb onto slippery roofs or scramble out of wrecked buildings into bobbing rescue boats. At times, like FDR, we may have to, or may even choose to, take a calculated risk and hope for the best. It's an individual call.

SO WHAT KEEPS US FROM GETTING STARTED?
WHAT WAS THAT CHAPTER ALL ABOUT?

The goal for us Seniors is to die young but as late as possible. And doctors say we can if we stay active. What fences in some Seniors is the fear of falling. The worst thing we Seniors can do is give in to irrational fears and stay inactive. We need to be willing to try to become more active. No one can make this decision for us.

But not all hazards are imaginary. It's not the big risks that lead to falls. It's the small risks that may trip us up. We have to use common sense—showing care and forethought.

Will this guarantee a future without falls? No. But we can sharply cut down the probabilities that we might fall. For us unsteady Seniors, calculated risks will be rare or nonexistent, but, at some time, they may present themselves.

Chapter 6

THE UNSTEADY SENIOR LISTS HIS
STEPPING STONES TO RECOVERY

Earlier, I noted that I grew up in Missouri, the "Show-me" state. The advice on balance I was willing to follow had to be based on professional scientific studies rather than someone's armchair notions.

When possible, I also tried out every recommendation to see if it worked for me. When I found something that passed this test, I called it a stepping stone to recovery. Below are those that helped me.

But when I read Don's chapters, I found that he also listed what I thought were my unique discoveries. So you get them twice. He also added one, which I now add to mine. But I still feel right and good about discovering and checking it all out for myself.

HOW RESEARCHERS SAY THAT WE NAVIGATE

People, the experts say, get balancing signals in three ways.

Vestibular signals. Those waving hairs in our inner ear send suggestions to our brains. This is our basic equilibrium. In Don's section, you'll find a simple way to test if your vestibular balance is okay.

If vestibular imbalance is a problem, it requires medical attention. It can be caused by migraines or an ear infection causing inflammation. More commonly, the cause is bits of calcium carbonate crystals that break down and collect within the semicircular canals.

Your ear, nose, and throat doctor will call what you have benign, paroxysmal positional vertigo (BPPV). That was put in just in case you want to understand what he or she and the nurse are talking about.

The doctor will likely prescribe some eye and motion exercises called Cawthorne's Head Exercises, Epley or Semont maneuvers, or Brandt-Daroff exercises. These are specific sequential movements designed to move the particles into an area of your inner ear where they can't affect balance, thus screening out false signals to your brain. But no refunds on this handbook because you'll soon be back.

Such exercises are, for example, focusing on a point while moving your head from side to side or walking while nodding or moving your head from side to side. Relief comes in four to ten weeks.

The International Vestibular Disorders Association is located in Portland, Oregon, and more information can be found at **www. vestibular.org/resources.html.**

Somatosensory directions. We already noted in the research chapter that messages are sent up to the brain through sensors or receptors at nerve endings, especially those at the bottom of our feet and also in our hands and other parts of our bodies. They get whisked upward through the central nervous system to the cerebellum.

Visual cues. What we see, supplemented by what we hear, also give us suggestions about how to navigate. These visual cues give us a sense of our position in space.

How We Unsteady Seniors Navigate

Assuming we unsteady Seniors have enough muscle strength to get around, we do our balancing mostly by letting our vestibular sense and our eyes guide us, plus sometimes adding in a little wild guesswork.

Generally, our vestibular signals are coming through okay, but they aren't sufficient by themselves.

STEPPING STONE TO RECOVERY 1: When our vision is blocked, we unsteady Seniors are heading for a fall.

For unsteady Seniors, visual cues are the major substitute for the garbled cues that they get from the sensors at the bottom of their feet. Recall how Dr. Tinetti found that the blocking of vision was a major cause of serious falls.

Remember the descriptions of my first three falls—carrying something down a stairs and couldn't see my feet, trying to navigate down a step at the cottage without looking down at where I was stepping, and going into a darkened room and getting tangled in computer wires.

They all showed a lack of commonsense, but what I didn't emphasize earlier is that they all occurred because I had blocked out those important visual cues.

When we are in the dark or in dim light or when our eyes are closed or we are blinded by glare from the sun, snow, or bright lights, even water splashing in our face in the shower, we unsteady Seniors are in danger of a slip and fall. Awareness of this is half the battle.

STEPPING STONE TO RECOVERY 2: Imaging, balance exercises done correctly, Tai Chi, and dancing all helping restore the muscle and reflex memories in our cerebellum and so helping us improve our balance.

Garbled muscle memories. Since accurate messages aren't getting sent up to headquarters from those nerve endings in the feet, we sometimes get confused about where our feet are located. Our nerve-based communication system has somehow gotten static.

What happens then is that patterns that our brain has stored away tend to get blurred. When the cerebellum no longer gets accurate signals, its memory of where those feet are begins to fade, and we get confused and equally important; we lose reflex memories.

Retraining our brains. Imaging, balance exercises, Tai Chi, and dancing, as the researchers have discovered, all have been found to change brain images. They correct muscle and reflex memories.

But I learned that we unsteady Seniors have to do the movements with precision. That is why the fixed routines of Tai Chi and ballroom dancing are so effective. We sway through a series of varied controlled movements, in which we shift our weight from one foot to another. Balance exercises are designed to do the same job.

STEPPING STONE TO RECOVERY 3: Light touch with a cane or a gently touch on walls adds to our position sense.

My brother-in-law, an orthopedist claims it is easier to get people to jump off the top of a building than to get them to use a cane. After I had a knee operation, he insisted I buy one of those sit-down ones, which I used for a while and then put aside. My surgeon tried a different approach on me. He started out, "Now, Charlie, you're an intelligent fellow, etc., etc." And my primary care physician, noting my unsteadiness, repeated the same refrain about using a cane.

The result was the same in all cases. I strongly resisted their suggestions. The way they all put it, it seemed to me that a cane would be the first step on the way to a walker and then a wheelchair.

The doctors didn't understand my obstinacy. They thought it was all vanity about looking old, though as Winston Churchill demonstrated, using a cane actually might make me look kind of distinguished, a real leap-forward fashion—wise for me.

Already, I had observed that when I used a cane on an airline or out on the town, I was treated with patience, kindness, and got help from strangers when struggling to get luggage out of the overhead bin or getting a seat on a bus. It gave me faith in the younger generation.

Still, I kept framing the cane question as a trade off-dependence versus independence. Only when I faced an especially questionable or new and potentially hazardous situation did I agree to put aside my pride and prejudices and take along a cane.

Then along came Don—the cane, he pointed out to me, was only to be used for light touching. It's a source of additional sensory data, giving us our position. It isn't supposed to hold us up.

Canes are like walls. Walls are also touchable. Touching keeps us walking straight rather than staggering along because we get accurate messages sent up to our cerebellums. This puts a whole new light on this cane thing.

Canes and walls are good friends.

Losing Our Balance

Webster's dictionary defines balance, as "an even distribution of weight ensuring stability."

The trouble is that we unsteady Seniors want to move about like other people, and that means we have to shift around the distribution of our weight. That calls for being temporarily off balance.

When we are inactive and stable, as in standing still, our center of gravity is directly over our legs, our base of support. When we move about, the trick is to go off balance and then make counter movements that shift our center of gravity back over our base of support. We thus have temporary periods of instability as we walk for example.

STRATEGIES FOR KEEPING OUR BALANCE

Everyone at times accidentally begins to lose his or her balance. The researchers say we then follow one of three strategies to keep from falling. All are attempts at getting our center of gravity back over our base of support.

The ankle strategy. This works for minor upsets. We unsteady Seniors shift our center of gravity backward or forward by rotating our body around the ankle joints to bring it back over the base of support. As an unsteady Senior, you may find yourself doing this while waiting in line or standing still for a long time.

The hip strategy. This helps avoid the more serious upsets. We move the hips one way or the other to regain balance. When we bend the knees to brushing our teeth or washing our hands, we are shifting the hips over our base of support. We may also find ourselves shifting our hips at more perilous times, as when we begin to tip side way or perhaps when we are temporarily blinded as in taking a polo shirt off over our heads.

The stepping strategy. This occurs when we stumble or are pushed backward. We take several quick steps forward to get steady.

STEPPING STONE TO RECOVERY 4: Strengthening our ankles, quadriceps, and our core muscles will help keep us from falling when we lose our balance.

These strategies are used to prevent falls by using our lower body muscles, especially ankle and leg muscles. Again, note Dr. Tinetti's discovery that muscle weakness is associated with falls, serious enough to cause a hip fracture.

Other research bears this out. The *Consumers Report on Health,* June 2007, states, "The ankles and thigh [quadriceps] muscles of frequent fallers were much weaker than those of similar nonfallers in a recent study of nursing home residents."

And researchers have found that walking does in itself markedly strengthens the quadriceps muscles. Researchers placed electrodes on the quadriceps and recorded electrical responses on individuals walking on level surfaces at a normal pace. The results revealed that the quad activity was minimal.

This doesn't mean we unsteady Seniors should give up walking as part of our exercise program. It is a good all-around exercise.

But we should not make it our sole exercise.

Help from the core muscles. Joseph H. Pilates, that early exercise pioneer, noticed that the core muscles, those that surround our bodies at the abdomen, transfer power to the extremities. This is why an amputee can walk when fitted with an artificial limb or a punter will use his whole body to get a really long kick.

These core muscles also give us extra strength to assist us when using any of the three strategies that keep us upright.

STEPPING STONE TO RECOVERY 5: Correct posture will help us unsteady Seniors maintain balance.

Already, I noted why the Leaning Tower of Pisa leans. It was not built perpendicular to the earth, and so gravity has been gradually pulling it down. The same is true of us. When we lean in any direction, we are challenging gravity.

As we grow older, many of us tend to lean forward. Check this out the next time you are at a mall. Notice how many Seniors do this. Then notice how seldom the younger set lean forward as they walk.

The unsteady Senior writing this regularly walks with a friend who does no other exercising. He is a great walker and can walk faster and much farther than me. But he likes to walk clasping his hands behind his back and leaning forward. He has fallen forward at least three times I know of, once even breaking his wrist.

We unsteady Seniors have to defy gravity to stay active. Stronger muscles can help us recover when we lean too far forward.

But is it wise to make a habit of leaning forward into a possible fall? Does it make sense to habitually defy gravity for no good reason?

STEPPING STONE TO RECOVERY 6: Keeping flexible is an important part of staying upright.

Those with arthritis need to extend their range of motion, and this is true of many of the sedentary as well as the rest of us when we reach that eminent Senior status. Stiffness can only be avoided by doing something about it.

Stretching exercises are helpful for all of us unsteady Seniors.

It is not clear that a stretching warm up will help us avoid injuring muscles when we exercise as was once thought. But for us unsteady Seniors, getting rid of stiffness and extending our range of motion by doing stretches does help us with our balance and thus reduce the probability of a fall.

STEPPING STONE TO RECOVERY 7: Unsteady Seniors need to eat a proper diet and not become grossly overweight.

This is the only one we have to take partly on faith, hoping the nutritionists know what they are talking about. They say that proteins are especially important for us Seniors. We already suspect that candy and donuts and potato chips are probably not the best as a steady diet.

But we do know what extra weight does to our knees

THE CONCLUSIONS THIS UNSTEADY SENIOR REACHED

For starters, unsteady Seniors need to check in with their doctors, especially the eye doctors. Then they need to be willing to try to become more active. And when facing risks, they need to use forethought and care, combining prudence and commonsense.

This strolling along on a series of stepping stones has taken us to a familiar destination, a program of posture, stretching, balance, and strengthening exercises, with a suggestion that we also follow a proper diet. Such a set of exercises designed for unsteady Seniors will be found in Don's section.

He also warns us to be careful not to block our vision and tells us why using a cane and lightly touching walls are helpful.

Now, at least, we know why we should be doing all these things to reduce the probability of a serious fall. And I, for one, find a measure of satisfaction in having gone through this process rather than just doing what the experts tell us to do.

It is not a good idea to blindly trust the experts. Sometimes when you just get the hang of something you have been working on for years, they do some more research and change their minds. It is good to test and check things out for yourself.

STEPPING STONES TO RECOVERY
WHAT WAS THAT CHAPTER ALL ABOUT?

Blocking our vision spells trouble. Tai Chi, ballroom dancing, and balance exercises properly done reactivate muscle and reflex memories in our brains. Canes and touching walls give us position sense lost because of those lazy sensors in our feet. Strong ankles, quadriceps, and core muscles keep us steady when we lose our balance. Correct posture and staying flexible also help. And a well-rounded diet and not becoming grossly overweight is helpful.

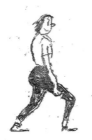
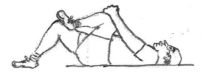

Chapter 7

The Unsteady Senior Shares Some Discoveries While Navigating

You may find a few of my discoveries helpful. As a personal reminder, I keep a short list of some of them in the back pocket of my exercise shorts. It is a helpful guide as I attempt to recall the good ideas that I intended to try.

Discovery Number One: Guiding Our Center of Gravity

Your center of gravity is located somewhere behind your belt buckle. That is at your navel, and I discovered a very useful thing. The center of gravity is affected by two extensions.

Anyone who has done a little carpentry knows that you can best make the hammer hit the nail on the head with full force if you hold the handle at the very end rather than close up to the shank.

In a way, our bodies are like two hammers with the claws meeting at the center of gravity. We have one extension from our center of gravity down to our feet and another that extends upward to our head.

We know how just a small movement at the ankle level affects our balance. The same must be true of small movements at the other end of our upper body.

Imagine one of the controls of balance being just below my chin and how I retain better balance by not tilting to the side. I steer with my shoulders while swinging my arms.

You will notice that tightrope walkers don't always hold their poles at the waist where the center of gravity is but sometimes seem to think it gives them better balance to hold them across the shoulders.

But then Don pointed out to me that the position of our head is what really affects balance. If we bend it over to one side, we tend to lose our balance in that direction. Notice that those tightrope walkers always look straight ahead, never to the side or down, lest they lose balance.

DISCOVERY NUMBER TWO: SPOTTING LIKE A BALLERINA

Earlier, I noted that another Senior told me that when you feel a little unsteady, it helps to concentrate on something that goes straight up and down, that is vertically.

Here are some tips along the same line from a former ballerina. If you notice, and I confess I never did, when these dancers spin, their heads whip around always to the same position. That's because they are concentrating on a distant spot and returning to that spot with every spin. This keeps them balanced and prevents dizziness.

You can maybe use this trick when doing various things. Just look away at eye height at something fifteen or so feet away and concentrate on that particular spot as you move around.

DISCOVERY NUMBER THREE: DOING THE STORK

The stork exercise is standing on one foot without holding on. This is an item that may make you feel better about your progress.

Jane Brody put this in a *New York Times* column on January 8, 2008. These are the norms for various age groups doing it for as long as possible.

20 to 49 years old:	24 to 28 seconds
50 to 59 years old:	21 seconds

60 to 69 years old: 10 seconds
70 to 79 years old: 4 seconds
80 and older: Can't do it at all

It's okay to settle with being as good as your age group, but perhaps you might want to strive to be like those above-average kids who inhabit Lake Wobegon. It's a good secondary goal!

DISCOVERY NUMBER FOUR: OUR UNAPPRECIATED BIG TOES

Here I'm really pioneering out on the cutting edge.

As we struggled with balance, we should became more aware of the way our big toes help steady us. They are not built like our other toes. They are of major importance when we do the rock-and-roll movements. They help push us forward when walking and also assist in stability when standing in place.

When I roll the soles of my feet slightly inward toward the big toes and inner heels, I feel more steady and more in control. I also tend to walk straighter rather than side to side. Depending on the little toe and the outer heel to do the job could be a disaster.

Let me warn you that I have never seen an article or heard any expert discuss the importance of big toes for balance or for anything else except that's where gout pain finds a real welcome.

DISCOVERY NUMBER FIVE: GETTING BOXED IN

One of my early falls happened when I tried to thread my way through boxes of clothes and other trash that my granddaughter had dumped on the floor in a back bedroom. All at once, I landed on my bottom. Nothing was hurt except my dignity. Lucky again!

What happened is that where I wanted to step next was covered with junk. I wobbled my foot around in air and then fell.

A condition we unsteady Seniors desperately have to avoid is getting our feet trapped so that the place we need to step next isn't blocked. This is how we lose our balance. In our younger days, this was less of a problem, but now we find ourselves toe dancing and reaching our foot out into the air and will most likely end up falling.

Like all of us, I knew that I'd fall if I got entangled in something like a vacuum cleaner cord or a garden hose. What I hadn't realized is that it was just as bad if I ventured into a place where the options of where I could step were limited.

We can get boxed in when we get our lawnmower out of the garage or shed and where gas cans, rakes, and cardboard boxes are all crowded together. We can even get boxed in by the clutter around our good old easy chair. Think about that!

DISCOVERY NUMBER SIX: STANDING IN LINE

One problem many of us unsteady Seniors face is occasionally standing still in a line or standing around in a crowd at a party making pleasantries without something or someone to hang on to. This is where a cane comes in handy.

My problem, I figured out, was weak ankles. Trying to do a toe lift on my weak foot was a joke, and I couldn't do the heel lift except when sitting down, not even when standing in water.

Early on, I had to develop some substitute strategies. Standing in place, I found I could balance most easily with my feet spread apart. Also, at first I found it helpful to hold my hands behind my back, much like the posture of a baseball umpire. As I now know, Don says that's a real no-no because we get in the habit of leaning forward.

Actually, as I've exercised, I found that I no longer need my arms behind my back for steadiness. It seems that by concentrating on the balls of my feet rather than my heels, I have better control—ankle balancing.

Bending my knees slightly also helps because it shifts my center of gravity over my base of support and also because the muscles in my legs are stronger than those in my ankles. It's probably not the best form a posture, but it's better than falling on my face, and I am exercising my ankles at the same time.

Once an orthopedic doctor told me the ankle opposite the knee operation gets weak. Have no idea if it's true.

DISCOVERY NUMBER SEVEN: CARRYING THINGS

Carrying anything means problems. We may be unable to see our feet or to grasp the railing. Using a cane is more difficult, and our hands can't as easily prevent or break a fall. Also it can just throw us off balance.

Balancing becomes tricky, regardless of how the items are held. Carrying requires an adjustment as our center of gravity moves more forward. Failure to adjust may cause us to stagger or lean forward. This is especially so if it's heavy. When we have to carry an object with only one hand, like a travel bag, the center of gravity shifts to that side.

It is probably best, when going upstairs, to put the package on the first step and to move it up one at a time. Going down is harder, but some things you can just slide down the steps without hurting anything, even when they make a crashing sound.

If we can put an item on wheels, it helps, as with luggage. At the cottage, I sometimes use a wheelbarrow or an icebox on rollers when bringing cartons of soft drinks and other bulky groceries from the car into the house.

The only other thing we can do is to be aware of the problem and be careful, or we can push such tasks on to others. Especially in airports, pay a red cap to do the job.

DISCOVERY NUMBER EIGHT: THINGS WE DROP

The American Academy of Orthopedic Surgeons says that when we stoop, we should bend our knees and squat and keep our back straight.

This will be a problem for Seniors with arthritis in the knees. Whether they want to or not, they may just find themselves leaning forward into a precarious balance because they can't bend knees enough to stoop all the way down. So hold on to something.

We Seniors have all noticed that when we drop something, it seems to get lost down there much more quickly than it used to. Things just roll away and hide. Let's just figure that the sneaky-floor monster that lives down there gobbled it up. If it's a really important item, or we are afraid of stepping on it, we can usually get someone else to crawl around to find it.

A friend told me this. If we do really have to stoop or kneel down, we might find it useful to look around for whatever else we can find while we're down there. You never know what you'll find.

One trick if you see the dratted object is to kick it over close to something steady you can hang on to while you reach down.

We get the same advice from the AAOS for lifting things. When we lift, we should put our feet shoulder width apart and be on solid ground. We should bend our knees, tighten our stomach muscles, squat down, take a firm grip, and lift with our knees rather than our back, keep our back straight, put our weight in our legs, and hold what we lift close to our bodies.

We should never lift while our back is twisted. My former partner in writing textbooks, Ken, recently told me he wrenched his back lifting something while bending sideways. Most of the rest of us have never been tempted to do anything so silly. Just kidding, Ken; he can take it.

DISCOVERY NUMBER NINE: HOLDING A CANE

We know we should only touch with our cane, but sometimes it helps momentarily to lean, and that can become a habit. You may settle for that as the status quo, but if not, hold the cane in your hand loosely and walk along for a bit. It may even help to reverse the handle in your hand while you are making it a habit again to only touch.

DISCOVERY NUMBER TEN: LENGTHENING OUR STRIDE

To lengthen your stride, strike the heel of your shoe with each step. You will walk faster and be less likely to catch a toe.

DISCOVERY NUMBER ELEVEN: THE WEAKER LEG

When walking, I noticed that I most often stepped to the side with my right foot. It took me a while to figure out that this was because my left foot and ankle were weak and needed special strengthening.

Non-discovery Number One: How to Play in Traffic

These aren't really discoveries and probably most of our generation has already figured these out, but here they are anyways. On roads without sidewalks or on country black tops, we are safer if we walk along on the edge, which would be the left lane. That way, we can see cars coming at us and take evasive actions if our reflexes are still intact.

Wearing bright colored or reflective clothing may also make us more visible. I would also like to think the car drivers can see us better if we are looking at them, but that doesn't make any sense.

Non-discovery Number Two: Changing Direction Suddenly

As long as we unsteady Seniors are walking straight ahead, we're usually okay. A problem may occur when we suddenly decide to change directions, reach up high for something, bend down, look backward over our shoulders, or step backward.

We lose our base of support as our full weight is transferred to only one foot while the other one is out of position to help. It is possible that we may be shifting our weight to a leg that is too weak to hold us up. An awkward position may be another challenge. We may end up like Charlie Chaplin taking his skip-hop around a corner.

If you have a suggestion for helping with the problem of sudden direction change, besides going into an exercise program that strengthens your leg muscles or doing balance exercises or Tai Chi, the rest of us unsteady Seniors would be glad to hear about it.

Some Discoveries for Navigating
What was that chapter all about?

Among the discoveries I've made were balancing with the upper body, using spotting, how long to do the stork, the usefulness of our big toes, not getting boxed in, help for standing in line, what to do when carrying or dropping something, to avoid locking my knees, walking on streets without curbs, and the problems of changing direction.

Chapter 8

The Unsteady Senior Makes Some Discoveries While Exercising

My First Discovery: The Importance of Form in Balance Exercises

As already noted, I began working on my balance situation pretty much on my own by exercising haphazardly. Then I brought Don into the act. I always wondered why physical therapists were so prissy about doing exercises so exactly.

Like many others, I've always been a little impatient. Getting it over with has sometimes been more important than getting it right. Until the reason was pounded in, I'd go ahead fast as I could.

Then came the discovery. No one told me about this. The literature I read didn't point this out. Maybe the writers thought it was self evident to everyone but a few klutzes like me.

The sun broke out from behind the clouds one day when I was going back over the research chapter. Balancing exercises, I realized, are supposed to retrain our cerebellum to help us Seniors regain the muscle memory as to where our feet are.

Here I was innocently trying to walk a straight line, heel to toe, and often tottering and staggering around to keep from falling down. The positional messages I was sending upstairs for filing were pretty much emphasizing the kind of motions I was hoping to erase. Talk about sending mixed messages.

This reminds me of the great jazz trumpeter, Bunny Berrigan, who played with Tommy Dorsey and Artie Shaw and later had a big band of his own. One day, he came weaving in, very tipsy, but somehow managed to climb up onto the bandstand and find his trumpet. Then off he went on his beautiful interpretation of "I Can't Get Started With You."

Someone later asked him how he could play so well given his bombed-out condition. "I'll tell you my secret," he answered. "I practice drunk."

The message my cerebellum was getting was a little as if I had been practicing while off on some kind of tear. Berrigan had the right idea; practice it the way you want it to come out so that the cerebellum gets the right messages to store away.

Walking heel to toe, you can hold on to the counter with one finger, and also you can when doing the stork, rather than flailing around trying to keep your balance.

The why of Tai Chi. One day, I got to wondering why Tai Chi was so helpful for balance. Then it came to me. Tai Chi is not a repetitive routine as many balancing and stretching exercises are. You have to follow along through various moves. You must concentrate on what comes next and be in control every minute.

Could we add more contrology to balance and stretch exercises? For those balance and stretch exercises where I can hold on to something, I found ways to make it more likely that I follow each movement, particularly as I emphasize the holds. I added some slow swings and carefully watched as I did them.

My Second Discovery: Sometimes Form Gets in the Way

You remember that old joke about the centipede? He got tied up in knots because someone asked him which foot he moved first when he started to walk.

Our goal is to adopt proper form without thinking about it. We can practice walking making sure we rock and roll, but when we take off onto the open road, it's a different story.

Just do it! Obsessing over technique can ruin performance. The same is true after you've established proper form in exercising.

That philosophical athlete, Yogi Berra, once observed, "you can't think and hit at the same time." You'll think yourself into a batting slump if you keep watching what you're doing all the time. When we're out walking, we want to do the right thing automatically without fussing about how to go about it.

When all we do is think about technique, we also take all the enjoyment out of a pleasant stroll around the neighborhood.

You could sing to yourself a cheerful song—say "Toot, toot, tootsie, goodbye. Toot, toot, tootsie, don't cry" or maybe "Hello my baby. Hello my honey. Hello my ragtime gal" to yourself, I suggest.

Or you could listen to books on tape for distraction and let your muscle memory take over.

My Third Discovery: The Value of Slowing Down

Most of the time when I started exercising seriously, I rushed along because I wanted to get the whole thing over quickly. What I had been doing, especially when daydreaming, was going at it like one of those arms on the side of an old-fashioned steam locomotive.

Bouncing—that's what trainers call it. This is what I was doing as I exercised: jerking back and forth and bouncing from one position to the other. Sometimes I still catch myself doing it. We are all probably natural born bouncers.

Bouncing makes the muscles tighten and even to the extent of straining them. Bouncing is one of those deadly sins, like eating Twinkies.

When bouncing, we are going through an exercise on built-up momentum—what the first George Bush called the Big Mo-wild swinging motions that let us coast along from the first push. These reckless swinging motions leave us pretty much out of control and let our muscles coast along without doing very much work.

You may be tempted to coast on momentum on the return or downswing of a strengthening exercise, letting gravity just take you along and then bounce back up when you get to "start." You may also depend on momentum if the weight you are using is too heavy for you to control except by giving a strong push and swinging up. Or you may tire doing a strengthening exercise, perhaps around eight reps, and begin bouncing. If you are doing one leg at a time, you can switch to the other leg and go to eight reps and then come back to the first leg and complete the set.

Just remember momentum is the enemy. Our muscles get less out of an exercise when we swing along and give the muscles a free ride. We lose all control and lapse into bad form and so lose some of the benefit of the exercise. *So slow down!*

Joseph Pilates called his exercise system *Contrology*. Exercise, to be helpful, he claimed, has to be done as a carefully controlled movement. That means slowing down and taking note. He suggests that we exercise, for want of a better word, *deliberately,* which the dictionary defines as "done consciously and intentionally, carefully and unhurried."

What I found out is that when I slowed down and controlled the movement, I had to put more effort into the exercise. Not surprising when you think about it since I was no longer letting the momentum do the work.

The first time I tried slowing down, I felt a little stiff the rest of the day. Those muscles really got a workout. Then I found I could reduce the repetitions or reduce the weights.

THE FOURTH DISCOVERY: HOW TO MAKE SURE TO SLOW DOWN

Control came most easily if I counted in a slower manner. You can slow down if you count one hundred and one, one hundred and two, etc. Or you can do one thousand and one. Sometimes, I've even done one million and one, when I wanted to feel I was getting somewhere.

Still, I've found what for me is another way to make sure I slow down and have a long-enough *hold* and a long-enough *rest* when I return to start. I repeat the number of the reps two times as one-one, two-two, etc.

It becomes a habit very quickly.

If you want try a go-slow program suited to us Seniors, do the one-one-one on the upswing, one-one-one on the hold, then one-one-one on the downswing, and finally one-one-one on the rest.

But I found when counting all those numbers, it sometimes would all run together. So I did one-one-one *clang* on the approach, one-one-one *ding* on the hold, one-one-one *clang* on the return, and one-one-one on the rest. Only later did I realize that "The Trolley Song" that Judy Garland made famous was where I got all those clangs and dings.

One of the advantages of this system is that even if your mind wanders, the clangs and dings go on without you thinking about it. Before, I would just start bouncing.

You might want to be more dignified and rational and do one-one-one up and one-one-one hold, one-one-one down, and end with one-one-one rest.

Another way I sometimes use is the old yell from hide and seek when we kids ran home free—Olly, olly, oxen, free, one.

A second way to slow down is to make sure that the *holds* are really *holds*. If you really hold while you count one-one-one *ding*, or whatever, you are half way on the road to stopping bouncing. The other half is to take a little rest break at *start*.

Just remember Gene Tunney. A slow, long count saved him when he was groggy in his championship fight with Jack Dempsey.

DISCOVERY NUMBER FIVE: THE SEVENTEEN STUMBLE

Sometimes, on a thirty-count stretch, I would sail along through the count and, at other times, stumble at *seventeen*. It took me a while to figure it out. It's because all the other numbers from thirteen to nineteen have a single syllable followed by "teen"—all except *se-ven-teen*. It throws off the rhythm. Just a bit of trivia you can use to impress someone about how serious you are about exercising.

DISCOVERY NUMBER SIX: WHEN YOUR MIND WANDERS

Like most of us, my mind sometimes wanders off now and then, thinking about why the Detroit Tigers and the Lions take nosedives and other such important matters.

It is useful, I've found, to start every exercise with the same foot, arm, or big toe and start off those motions going clockwise. Then if your mind flies off thinking about MSU and the March Madness and suddenly comes back to what's going on, you know where you are in the routine by checking which foot you're on.

If you want to check how long you walked, you have to remember when you started. That isn't always easy for some of us. Tie the number to something, especially something odd. If it's 21 to the hour, remember it as "twenty-one ski doo," though we Seniors know that's not exactly the way it goes. If it's ten after, think ten pins. If it's twelve to two, that old time movie actress, Helen twelve trees. If it's thirteen to, then Helen thirteen trees. Unless you walk for two hours, you should be able to remember whether you started "to" or "after" the hour, all on your own.

DISCOVERY NUMBER SEVEN:
THE IMPORTANCE OF WRITING IT DOWN

After a while, I checked the list of exercises I was doing. And what do you know? I was leaving one out. A Senior moment? Not really. I just caught myself committing a little sloth.

Some of us, including me, seem to forget parts of exercises or even whole exercises that we don't like very much or find a little boring. We may even catch ourselves working out illegal shortcuts. I keep a short list in the back pocket of my gym shorts, and when it seems the exercises are going too fast, I've consult it; and once or twice, what do you know?

Most of you unsteady Seniors are probably not like that at all, but still it won't hurt anything for you to look over the list every month or so. Checking every so often also lets you add or subtract one or more exercises.

DISCOVERY NUMBER EIGHT:
BREATHING WHILE EXERCISING

At first I had trouble with this. Even sometimes I caught myself holding my breath. The reason we shouldn't hold our breath while doing exercises, Don tells me, is that it deprives our body of needed oxygen and will increase blood pressure temporarily.

Finally, I began to train myself to exhale slowly going forward on an exercise, inhale on the hold, exhale on going back, and inhale at rest. It will slow you down a little too.

This puts the exhaling during the straining part of an exercise and inhaling in between the rests. The straining part is when we are most tempted to hold our breath. We also may hold our breath, I've found, when we do those stretching exercises. Those are the ones where we have to count to thirty.

DISCOVERY NUMBER NINE: NOT OVERDOING IT

As I have been told, I sometimes get a little impatient. Several times, I've had the idea that when something is working, it would work twice as fast if I doubled the weights or the reps. *Dumb idea!*

Once, I increased a leg weight more than I should have, or I did too many repetitions. I forget which. For my overzealousness, I got some real muscle pain that lasted a couple days.

Worse than that, I once did too many repetitions of a stretching exercise and ended up limping around with a cane, and this time it was helping hold me up. This lasted four or five days. Nance and I had a luncheon date with another couple. We had to go since we already cancelled out once before.

As I struggled with a cane on a long walk across a relatively deserted restaurant to our table, I could feel everyone's eyes on me. The waitresses seemed ready to rush over and catch me, but I made it by myself, only just barely. Everyone, including me, gave a sigh of relief. My friends were probably surprised when after a week or so, I could walk more normally again.

Also, I found that when I overdo it even just a little, I seem to get more unsteady.

So easy does it. Just listen to what your body is whispering or maybe even shouting at you. Hurrying just makes things go longer.

DISCOVERY NUMBER TEN: DOING FUNCTIONAL EXERCISES

Herm Schneider, the White Sox trainer who I mentioned earlier, says he tries to give his players functional exercises—those that are similar to the kinds of actions he is trying to improve.

For us Seniors, getting up out of a chair is such a functional exercise. So too are many of the balance exercises. If you have a choice, go functional.

DISCOVERY NUMBER ELEVEN:
THE BEST EXERCISE EQUIPMENT

You will get more use out of a set of those rubbery exercise stretch bands than almost any piece of equipment you can buy. They are cheap; you can use them anywhere, at home or on vacation; and they come in different strengths according to their color. The ones I bought use this color coding system. Don tells me others may vary in their color codes.

Extra light	Peach
Light	Orange
Medium	Green
Heavy	Blue
Extra heavy	Plum

DISCOVERY NUMBER TWELVE:
IF YOU HAVE TO TAKE A BREAK

Life is so unpredictable that interruptions in our exercise routine are inevitable. These can be because of illness or injury, entertaining out of town friends, or holiday festivities.

Taking a few days or weeks off because we don't feel like exercising isn't on the list.

On vacation. What is most upsetting to routines is a change of location. That's because we have to fit in a whole new time for exercising and maybe even a new routine because we can't drag along a set of dumbbells, and, besides, we don't want to be doing the stork in front of friends.

We Seniors on vacation are also somehow likely to eat more (Hey, it's vacation.) and exercise less, except for walking.

Somehow we need to fit as much of our exercise routine into the chaos of each new day. Even if we feel we deserve a break, we can still fit in a little. The one piece of equipment easy to pack is the rubbery exercise stretch band. So we Seniors do the best we can and figure walking more makes some difference.

But despite the chaos, we know of two other daily routines we never duck out of. They remain unchanged even while on vacation—one is stretching when we open our eyes and wake up, and the other is just after we get into our pajamas and get ready to climb into bed. In each case, we can maybe squeeze in a few minutes of exercise but maybe not anytime after midnight or before 10:00 a.m.

The three-week rule. When we stop exercising, in about three weeks, the experts say we lose whatever strength we have gained. It will take us about nine weeks of exercising to get back to where we were, which doesn't seem quite fair.

And to add to our difficulties, our weight may also begin to creep up. Yet if we exercise only once a week, it helps us keep our gains.

Getting back into it. After a break in the routine, we need to restart slowly, perhaps reducing weights and repetitions. But the important thing is that we shouldn't let feelings of guilt keep us from getting back into the routine.

DISCOVERY NUMBER THIRTEEN:
IF YOU JOIN A HEALTH CLUB

If your lock doesn't have a distinctive look, put some whiteout on the edges of it, so you can spot your locker easily, and if you leave it behind one day, it's also easy to pick it out in the box of lost locks.

In the relaxation whirlpool, do the ankle lifts that you may not be able to do on dry land. Exercising in the dry sauna lets you see what you are doing, as the steam room does not. You may want to dispense with the large sports bag, dress at home, and put changes in a cloth shopping bag. It's easier to carry.

DISCOVERY NUMBER FOURTEEN: A PEDOMETER

Researchers at the University of Colorado found that using a pedometer added two thousand more steps daily (about a mile), prevented weight gain, and resulted in more physical activity.

If you want to get into this, get a good pedometer. The cheap ones you get for free don't work too well. Make sure to attach it on your belt loop or you are almost certain to have it drop off some time or other. It happened twice to me before I learned.

The *Journal of the American Medical Association* found that those of us who use pedometers also have a decrease in blood pressure. They found those who used them for eighteen weeks also increased to between 2,183 and 2,491 steps per day.

DISCOVERY NUMBER FIFTEEN: ONE FOOT AT A TIME

Some of us find that one foot is weaker than the other. When you exercise both feet at the same time, you may find, as I did, that the stronger one is doing most of the work while the weaker one coasts. So I began doing exercises one foot at a time, and sometimes I did more reps with the weaker foot.

DISCOVERY NUMBER SIXTEEN: PROGRESS

My experience has been that arm muscles are the easiest to build up. After what seems like only a short while, you can begin to feel those muscles bulging on your upper arm, just by pressing them with your thumb like you used to do as a kid.

The thigh muscles, quadriceps, and hamstrings, take longer to build up. But you can begin to feel their strength as you find you walk better with fewer lurches, and when you begin to lose your balance, you recover more quickly.

The ankles, I've found, take a lot of work to build up. Exercises like doing lift ups or doing a kind of hula seem to help. And if your ankles are really weak, you can do lift ups in a relaxation pool as starters.

DISCOVERY NUMBER SEVENTEEN: REMEMBERING THOSE MUSCLES

I find it helps sometimes when I exercise to put my mind on the muscle I'm stretching or strengthening. Slowing down and actually feeling the exercise hit the muscle down deep make it seem like I'm getting somewhere. Closing your eyes while feeling the muscle stretch or strengthen also helps.

Also, when you just loosen up, say moving your ankle back and forth, take a tip from the ART practitioners (chapter 3) and put some muscle into it at the same time.

DISCOVERY NUMBER EIGHTEEN: SOURCES OF INFORMATION

The internet now provides more information than any reasonable person can absorb. But here are two sources of special interest to unsteady Seniors.

For more on balance, go to the website of the National Institute on Aging at http://nihseniorhealth.gov/exercise/toc.html and choose "Exercises for Older Adults," and then click on "Balance Exercises." Or call 1-800-222-2225 for a free copy of its "Exercise Guide," or purchase their exercise video or DVD.

The American College of Sports Medicine, June 1998 issue, had a series on exercise and physical activity for older Americans. The full text, which is concise but comprehensive, can be found on their website, *www.acsm.org.*The text is keyed into over 150 research articles listed as appendices.

Health letters. Seniors might find notes on balance problems from time to time in the many medical health letters. Among those available are those of the Mayo Clinic, the Cleveland Clinic, and the medical schools of Johns Hopkins, Harvard, the University of California, UCLA, Duke, and Tufts and of the Mount Sinai Hospital. Also, occasionally having such items are the *Consumer Reports on Health*, the *Center for Science in the Public Interest* reports, and news of research findings in the Tuesday "Science Times" of the *New York Times*. There are lots to choose from.

SOME DISCOVERIES WHILE EXERCISING
WHAT WAS THAT CHAPTER ALL ABOUT?

Topics covered: doing exercises haphazardly sends garbled messages on position sense up to the cerebellum, concentration on form can sometimes be counterproductive, why slow down and stop bouncing, how you count can help slow you down, tricks for getting back into the routine when your mind wanders, the importance of records, the seventeen stumble, proper breathing while exercising, not overdoing it, that the best kinds of exercises mimic things we do every day, when you have to take a break, the most useful equipment purchase you can make, tips if you join a health club, pedometers, exercising the weaker foot, and sources of further information.

Chapter 9

THE UNSTEADY SENIOR TACKLES

SOME DISCOVERIES FOR KEEPING AT IT

The American Cancer Society says the common excuses for not exercising are "I'm too busy," "I'm too tired," or "It's boring."

These pretty much boil down to the two related problems facing exercisers: "How can I be sure to keep at it?" and "How can I keep from getting bored?" We'll deal with keeping at it in this chapter and how to keep from getting bored in the chapter that follows.

YOUR OWN SPECIAL TRAINER

The best way to keep at it is to be under the care of a physical therapist or to hire a trainer from a health club, the way Hollywood movie stars do. They will ride herd on you to make sure you do all of the exercises and do them correctly, and they will encourage you.

Medicare pays for a certain amount of physical therapy, but you pay for the health club trainer. Most of us are probably not rich enough to employ a trainer.

Sooner or later, you have to recognize that most or all of the time, for the rest of your life, you will be the only special trainer you will ever have. No one else will be around to ride herd.

I'm afraid all of us, when it comes to exercising, all too easily adopt the phrase our youngest son thought was so useful as he was growing up. "Later, Mom, later!" (It didn't work.)

Somehow we alone have to figure out a way to get past "I'm too busy right now" along with all those other fine excuses.

A Role Model for All of Us Seniors

In *Newsweek* on September 26, 2005, Thomas Withers described an exercise program he wisely began when he was in his late forties. For thirty-seven years, he bicycled for ten miles, walked three miles, or climbed the stairs of a ten-story building five days a week.

He said he took fewer pills than his cat since he doesn't take any pills at all. He recently had participated in an annual ten-kilometer race. He came in first in the eighty-to-ninety-age category but also last at the very same moment. This tells us a little about sloth among the rest of the Seniors in his neighborhood.

For his magazine photo, he wore one of those wild floral sport shirts that we associate with Hawaii types, which tells us how much he was enjoying life to the fullest at age eighty-six.

Thomas Withers told the readers his secret of why he was now so healthy: *perseverance.*

Okay, so how do we get so that we persevere?

We Unsteady Seniors Already Have a Goal

An article in the *New York Times*, July 6, 2006, with headline: "Once an Athletic Star, Now an Unheavenly Body," Jill Agostino interviewed jocks who had been sport MVP's and VIP's in high school and college.

We nerds remember how they used to strut around flaunting their letter sweaters with a cheerleader on each arm. She now found a good many had gone to seed or just got plain fat (one five foot eleven was now topping 265). Many no longer were involved in any physical activity besides turning on the TV to shout valuable suggestions at other performing athletes.

Here is what one said, "I find it hard to get out there. There's nothing to shoot for." Tom Raedeke, associate professor of Sport Science at East Carolina University in Greenville, NC, said of these ex-athletes, "Exercise just seems to lack purpose or meaning. It's pointless." Without the goal of winning a game or showing off in front of those coeds sighing and cooing on the sidelines, it seems like a waste of time.

Unlike these ex-athletes, we do have an important goal to motivate us, to lead an active life while sharply reducing the probability of falling; so far so good.

A secondary goal. But that's not enough. It's too vague and general. We now need to have a specific secondary goal to aim for. It has to be simple and measurable so exercising can seem interesting and worthwhile.

That's what Thomas Withers did. His overall goal was to keep healthy, and he committed himself to exercising every weekday. His secondary goal was to cycle a certain distance every day or to do one of two alternate activities.

Franklin Roosevelt had the goal of being able to walk again. (You're right, I have a thing about how FDR handled being crippled and achieved so much.)

He discovered that he and other polio victims could do things in water they couldn't do on dry land, and so he began to swim every day. When he started, he found he could only stand in water up to his chin without his legs buckling. Then after many daily swims, the measure moved to the top of his shoulders, and finally, when he gave up the program to run for governor of New York, he was standing in water that reached under his arms.

His being able to stand in more and more shallow water kept him going. He could see he was making measurable progress toward his overall goal of being able to walk.

Our secondary goal might be to do fifteen or more seconds on one foot without holding on. When we have achieved this, we might next increase our ability to do a second set of reps of toe lifts. Walkers can time themselves over a certain distance and work at reducing the time it takes or walk farther in the same number of minutes.

We have to keep working out a continuing series of secondary goals to keep us going and show ourselves we are progressing.

So what's the next step?

Daily exercise does it. We know that part of achieving any of these secondary goals, as Thomas Withers shows, is daily practice, just like when some of us Seniors, way back then, started piano lessons. It was our mom, or knowing we'd have to face the teacher next week, that made us practice. We just knew that lady would tell our mom if we hadn't practiced and then it would come, "Why are we paying good money, and you don't even . . ."

We can't exercise just whenever we feel like it. Pretty soon, we'll forget all about the whole thing.

Then there's that other big danger point. The first time, we may have to skip a day. Will we ever get back again and keep going? When we pass this crisis, we Seniors can give ourselves a little pat on our back. But we need more than this to come back strong the next time a skipped day pops up.

How to keep at the daily exercising. Some twenty-one thousand readers were surveyed by the *Consumer Reports* magazine. They isolated the group who had a history of exercising for five years or more and asked them how on earth they kept at it so long.

They found a single characteristic that distinguished this group.

They exercised every day at the same time and also at the same place. *A specific time at the same place everyday*—that's what they said kept them at it.

When they skipped a day, these respondents said they felt somehow uncomfortable, vaguely uneasy. Something was missing.

Tie-ins to other rituals. It helps if you can tie your exercise routine into one of your other daily routines.

Most of us are retired, so we have more control over our daily lives. We can spend ten or so minutes stretching when we wake up in the morning and are still in bed. Nance and I do this.

I do an ankle strengthener right before I brush my teeth, along with a stork balance. I do this because I have weak ankles. I could just as well do this just before breakfast, but I don't. You could do strengthening exercises when you watch the evening news. Or take a daily walk every day an hour or so after lunch.

One of my sons is a former college and Olympic wrestler. He still works at his job, so evenings are the best time to can fit in exercising.

When visiting recently, I found he keeps in shape by doing a series of exercises every night while he watches an hour-long evening news program. It's a routine that his wife and kids expect and accept.

We can pick and choose a few special times or just one time. We don't have to turn into a perpetual motion, exercising phenomenon all day long. There are other things to do with our time.

But avoid certain times. These vary with the individual. Each of us unsteady Seniors have times when we'd rather be doing something else.

Some of us enjoy reading in bed before we go to sleep. Try as I have, I've never felt like fitting in an exercise then. If I try to schedule exercises as I'm getting into bed, I find myself torn, particularly when I see Nance already deep into a book.

I'm like the kid who was supposed to practice the piano while the kids outside called to come and play cork ball. I wanted to find out what happened next in that detective story, so I tried to get the exercises over as soon as possible and rushed through them and didn't do them very well, if at all. So I don't exercise at bedtime.

Strengthening exercises at home using strap-on weights are probably best done when watching TV, as my son does. It doesn't take extra time. Remember, it is easy to find any little excuse for not putting on the weights when you would rather be doing something else. Choose you designated time wisely so you can stick to it and still not interfere with your social life.

A Daily Log

At Health Clubs, the trainers keep track of every exercise they put you through. That's not a bad idea for unsteady Seniors to do as well, a daily check-off list.

My father wrote down his weight every morning in a little notebook. He took a lot of kidding about this in the family, but I guess it helped him keep off the weight. He thought so.

An alternative is to tack a chart up on the wall. It may seem a little showy, but it is intimidating. Crossing off the exercises every day will give you a feeling that you're making progress, and the blank spaces will send you off on a guilt trip. No one likes to see white among all those fine cross marks.

For the really busy, and aren't we all. Who said you have lots of leisure in retirement? Not someone already retired. If you keep a running date book, you might, just as important CEOs do, schedule in your exercise sessions. Or you could have your secretary jot it in for you. Just kidding.

A MOTIVATIONAL LIST

Daniel Stettner, a health psychologist at the Northpointe Health Center in Berkeley, Michigan, suggests that we unsteady Seniors paste on our bathroom mirrors a list of the benefits we are getting out of exercising. He calls it a daily motivator.

If you like that sort of thing, go for it. Here's some suggestions for your list.

The *Journal of Aging and Physical Activity* reports that 50 percent of decline between the ages of sixty and ninety-four could be alleviated through regular participation in moderate-level physical activity.

But they would say that, wouldn't they?

Still there's probably something to it. We'd better be on the safe side and get to that moderate physical activity, which for us is doing exercises and some walking. We can figure out the correct percentage of decline we stop in its tracks at some later date.

To add one little bit of inspirational information, the *Journal of the American Geriatric Society* reported that women who lifted weights for six months, did agility activities like dancing, ran obstacle courses, or did stretching exercises still benefitted from these activities a year later and reduced their chance of falls.

So there we have it, another item for our motivational list. But watch so you don't take a spill on that obstacle course. Why would anyone who runs obstacle courses worry about being unsteady?

SUPPORT FROM A FELLOW UNSTEADY SENIOR

We also may find it helpful to have someone else to work on the program with us, say a spouse, friend, or relative. Two women in our neighborhood walk the same route every day. If each did it alone, she might be tempted to skip or maybe stop altogether.

It takes character to our walk by ourselves, but when we know someone else is depending on us to show up, we feel we should also be there. These women always seem to be happily chatting away, so there's another side benefit.

Getting into an ongoing group is also good, for example those troops of mall walkers or groups at a Senior center. When choosing a walking partner, make sure they are motivated too. You wouldn't want a companion to draw you away from the exercises you should be doing.

For those who prefer getting their encouragement more impersonally, automated computer phone calls now exist that will nag you to exercise. The inventors say they are especially effective with Seniors who may feel intimidated by a trainer or even the fellow exercisers in their group.

COUNTING THE WEEKS

You may find it great on Fridays to count the weeks you've been at it. You'll be surprised how quickly they add up. It gives you a real kick to feel you're taking charge of this unsteadiness thing.

And as the weeks go by, you may want to add a little variety and change some of the exercises. A study at the University of Florida-Gainesville found variety adds to enjoyment and has the added benefit of helping people keep at it.

AND IF WE GET DISCOURAGED

We all get down at one time or another and think we aren't getting anywhere. One of our friends had a serious operation. During the recovery period the physical therapist had her doing over two hours of exercise a day. That included thirty-six minutes on the treadmill. I asked why the extra six minutes. She said it was in case she missed a day now and then; it would add up to an hour.

Her husband told me that almost every week she felt she wasn't getting anywhere. Yet each week when the physical therapist took measurements of her progress and found steady improvement.

We're all like that, I suppose. We expect to see spectacular and dramatic changes right now and get discouraged when it's incremental progress and not very much seems to be happening. That's why any kind of built-in measurement helps us keep at it.

Negative thoughts have a way of creeping back in, especially around the sixth to eighth week of exercising. At such down times, we just have to keep going.

So take the expert's word for it. You are improving and will improve more if you keep at it. Stop rattling around in all those clanking chains that hold you back, and, in case that lock seems somehow to have snapped shut again, grab that key and use it. Aren't those words of some kind of rock song?

THE PSYCHOLOGICAL HURT OF A FALL

We all know what happens if we take a fall. It's a sickening feeling. You have to be pretty much of a Pollyanna to smile happily and rise and shine. We'll rise, but we won't shine.

We may only be a little shaken up. But like soldiers after a skirmish, we can be hit later with a kind of post traumatic stress, and I'm not just kidding about this. I've been there. A feeling of "what's-the-use" sweeps over us; it seems like it shouldn't happen, but it does.

Almost everyone including the old whoopee Senior geezer writing this thing has experienced this sense of "Am I really getting anywhere?" But then we face the question of what will we do about it.

One psychologist says we should look at a fall as an opportunity to learn more about ourselves and why we fell. I suppose so. I've done a lot of thinking about the falls I've achieved all on my own, but it's not much of an upper.

Then there's the old song that says to just pick ourselves up and start all over again, and that's about it. At this stand, we won't hand out any other magic formula. We know we just have to keep going. Just remember we've all been through this and may have to face it again. We just have to keep going.

Just imagine the rest of us unsteady Seniors are all sympathizing with you, and we'll expect your sympathy when it's our turn.

BURNOUT

Trainers have found that burnout generally results by trying to do too much all at once. This is especially true for beginners who want to get right at it and solve all their difficulties right now.

Michael P. Maina, associate professor of Health and Human Performances of Roanoke College in Salem, Virginia, concludes that anyone who exercises more than an hour a day is probably overdoing it. His advice is "Take time, do less, but keep leaving it [your exercising] hungry every time, and you'll come back."

KEEPING A POSITIVE ATTITUDE

One study found Seniors with a positive attitude were more likely to begin and stay with an exercise program. Why wouldn't they? If you approach doing your exercises feeling you are gaining in strength and steadiness, you are more likely to keep going. If you start out pessimistic, it's easy to ask yourself, "Why am I torturing myself when I could be loafing in my easy chair sipping a cool sugary drink?"

Positive thinkers. You probably thought that the first positive thinker was the Rev. Norman Vincent Peale. But way back in 1909, Thomas Troward was pushing happy thinking in his *Edinburgh Lectures on Mental Science.* He worked out in a system where we begin with what we want and after a series of steps we end up imagining it will happen.

Troward said this way back then, "Those who say 'I can' and those who say 'I can't' are both right." Sometimes you might want to hit him.

And of course there's Johnny Mercer with "You gotta ac-cen-tu-ate the pos-i-tive."

The positive thinkers say that we should not look at our exercise program as a chore or duty, not using downer words as "I should" or "I ought" or "I must." We should use such positive words as "I want to," "I feel like," or "It'll help me to" or "I can handle it."

Just don't say these things out loud when strangers are around. Whatever works for you, Mercer, Peale, Troward, or Coue. If it helps, go to it. Try to think positively about this balance business when you can. It'll keep you at it.

Just so you know, one of those motivation guys measured all this. He said it takes about two weeks of hard practice to "e-lim-i-nate the neg-a-tive." So good luck.

Keeping It Pleasant

The stage actress and singer Kitty Carlyle Hart said that every morning, just before she did her exercises, she smiled at herself in the mirror. You might want to add a friendly "hi there!" and a wink!

My wife and I saw Ms. Hart on stage when she was in her early nineties. She tripped out in high heels, energetic and outgoing, smiled and sang, stood there, and talked for about fifteen minutes or more. She continued this routine up to six months before she died at age ninety-six, of heart failure.

So maybe there's something to this wearing a happy face.

Some Discoveries for Keeping at It
What was that chapter all about?

We unsteady Seniors have a goal which is to stay active while sharply reducing the probability of falling. We next need a series of secondary exercise goals as we achieve one and go on to another.

Researchers find that those who continue exercising over long period of years do so every day at the same time and the same place. If you are retired, you can more easily control the time you exercise.

It's helpful to tie exercising into one or more other daily routines. But avoid times when you may be cross pressured because you want to do something else. It is also helpful to keep a log and you may want to paste inspirational messages on your mirror.

All of us at one time or another get discouraged, especially so if we have a fall. We have to just pick ourselves up and keep going. Remember we all sympathize with you and we expect your sympathy when it comes to be our turn.

Those who can maintain a positive attitude are more likely to stick at an exercise program. It helps to keep a happy face.

Chapter 10

THE UNSTEADY SENIOR TACKLES

SOME DISCOVERIES FOR NOT GETTING BORED

They put TVs in front of treadmills at health clubs for a good reason. The repetitive treadmill walk gets pretty boring pretty quickly. So here from various sources are some suggestions on other ways to keep from getting bored.

A favorite program may remind us "Hey guys, it's that enjoyable exercise time!" But TVs are two edged. They may keep us going but also may distract us from watching what we're doing.

THE IMPORTANCE OF VARIETY

When you do the same routine over and over, your body begins adapt to it. The result is you get less and less benefit out of the exercise and studies have shown you even lose fewer calories. Doing something that uses different muscles actually improves the effect of your exercising as well as reducing boredom and the possibility of dropping out.

Susie Dashow, the general manager of a Seattle fitness club, recommends changing routines at least every six weeks.

Occasionally change the weights, the reps, the exercises, the rest periods, the incline on a treadmill, and anything else except for the time and place. You can change the order in which you do exercises if that doesn't mix you up so you leave out a couple. That may be why

Thomas Withers gave himself the choice of three activities, so none would bore.

You can reverse the counting of the reps. Ashley Borden, Nike spokeswoman, suggests that, instead of counting one to ten occasionally, we count backward as ten, nine, eight, etc. She says it will give us a feeling we're heading toward a finish line.

Joan Pagano has exercises available on a deck of cards. You can surprise yourself by pulling out a different set of exercises each day. Or you can make your own cards, but don't tell her I suggested it.

DOING IT WITH MUSIC

Jane Fonda does her exercises to music and many others have found this helpful. There is even an expert on this.

Costas Karageorghis, an associate professor of Sport Psychology at Brunel University in England, says when doing aerobic exercises for the heart, you should find music with a beat of 120 per minute, since that comes pretty close to the heart rate. He suggests "Drop It Like It's Hot" by Snoopy Dog or "Push It" by Salt-N-Pepa. So how about that? Don't ask me. Those unforgettable melodies are news to me too.

There's also on the market an MP3 player called Yamaha Bodibeat that scans your music collection and picks out melodies in sync with your heartbeat.

Feverish rock-and-roll or even Sousa marches may be a little over the top for us, unsteady Seniors. "The Blue Danube" or the slower rhythms of good old Glenn M. are probably more our speed, even if we prefer Fats Waller or Tommy Dorsey's Clambake Seven when loafing in our easy chairs.

BECOME A CULTURED TYPE WITH RECORDED BOOKS

You'll be amazed how many recorded books you can go through during the daily exercising. As a kid, I never really read *Robinson Crusoe*, though I once won a condensed version as a Sunday school prize. Recently, I went through the long version, the whole eight tapes. Honestly, but it was touch and go for a while. So I don't recommend that one.

Try P. G. Wodehouse. He's more fun. Or *A Tree Grows in Brooklyn*. But note, when I got deeply involved in this one, I forgot to go slow and even skipped whole exercises. That Betty Smith tale grabs you. Still, for me, listening to books and even old radio programs like "Lum and Abner" or Jack Benny makes the exercising all go by in a breeze. I even listen to old tapes of Hazen Schumacher's "Jazz Revisited Request Night" from that other university in Michigan.

Talking To Our Higher Selves

Murmurs, chants, shouts, and songs. Maybe you'll find giving sing-song messages to yourself helps so long as it doesn't end up as "Drill, Baby, Drill!" Even counting in rhythm can be helpful.

But I had enough of hup-two-three-four in the army, count off, etc. But there must be a reason drill sergeants do this sort of thing and sometimes get the ranks singing, "Oh the coffee that they give you, they say is mighty fine. It's good for cuts and bruises and tastes like iodine. Oh I don't want no more of army life. 'Oh Ma, I wanna go. Gee Ma, I wanna go. Oh Ma, I wanna go home.'"

In marching eight hours a day in basic, it seemed to me I was asleep or almost so as I heard those cadences. And they did help somehow. Anyhow, there were five minute breaks every hour. You can probably think up better stuff to tell yourself.

Now Nance says she does the grocery list while swimming. One day, she came back with the horrible information that we almost forget one of our grandkids' birthdays.

Or you can recite inspirational poetry to yourself that you learned in school: "Behind him lay the gray Azores," "I think that I shall never see a poem as lovely as a tree," or "Four score and seven years ago."

We Can Occasionally Reward Ourselves

We'll each have to figure out our own reward for the progress we make. Just don't make it too caloric.

One woman put a new dingle-dangle on her charm bracelet every time she met a specific goal.

JUST LET'S NOT GET TOO GRIM ABOUT THE WHOLE THING

Way back in the 1960s, the journalist and author Norman Cousins came down with Akylosing Spondylitis. (You could look it up.) The doctors gave him a fifty-to-one chance of recovery. He decided to check that old bromide that laughter is the best medicine. He isolated himself in a room all day and watched videos of "Candid Camera" and movies of the Marx Brothers, Laurel and Hardy and then, for some variety, read books and articles full of humor.

Besides the laugh routine, he also took vitamins and kept on a healthy diet. To his doctor's amazement, he cured himself. Then he wrote a book about it and began lecturing at medical conventions for a handsome fee.

Numerous research studies followed, all illustrating the benefits of laughter on various diseases and especially to control pain.

Maybe you won't be laughing your way through all your exercise routines (though you can find some pretty funny things on CDs and tapes). Still, just a cheerful outlook and an occasional joking around with other exercisers will make it more fun and make it more likely you'll stay with your program.

BOREDOM WHILE WALKING

Walking is a pleasant experience all on its own. However, some need more to keep them interested, so I pass along information on mindful and meditational walking.

Meditation walking. Meditation while walking follows the same principle as standing still meditation, breathing, concentration, and relaxation. The difference is that it's all combined with rhythmic slow walking. As you walk, you recite a mantra, but each of us unsteady Seniors will have to find his or her own; no one's passing out ready-made samples.

Mindful walking. This technique requires you to become aware of everything you are doing as you walk along, how the breeze feels, how your foot hits the pavement, how hard or soft the ground is, the chirping of birds, etc., etc. Doesn't sound like too bad an idea.

SOME DISCOVERIES FOR NOT GETTING BORED
WHAT WAS THAT CHAPTER ALL ABOUT?

One sure fire method for fighting boredom is to introduce variety in how you do the exercises, including even changing them from time to time.

You can add music and song, chants, or talking books. You can even have conversations with your higher self. But the main thing is, don't make everything too grim.

When walking, you can meditate or become aware of everything around you and what you are doing.

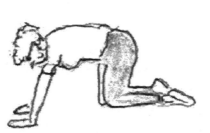
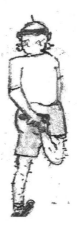

Chapter 11

THE UNSTEADY SENIOR REVIEWS
PRECAUTIONS WHILE MOVING ABOUT

Almost every so-called expert who writes about balance or falling and can't think of anything else to say to guide us unsteady Seniors lists things around the home that we might want to fall over.

Some ideas are pretty wild. I remember one with a picture that suggested we unsteady Seniors shouldn't leave our skateboards lying around in the front room.

The next chapter is about those homebound hazards. That's the easy part. Anyone can suggest we add a few safety gadgets like snapping a night light into a bath room plug. And you've probably heard of most of them and done something about them.

But to change how we unsteady Seniors navigate is much more difficult. It means breaking old habits.

So let's get on with how we unsteady Seniors can navigate and can avoid what spells trouble.

The experts have come up with some suggestions and some have popped up from my or the experiences that other unsteady Seniors have shared. Some of this advice may strike you as quite sensible. Other bits you may think are otherwise.

You'll have to sort this out for yourself.

GENERAL GUIDELINES

Get scared of the dark again. Let there always be light.

Wherever you step should be firm. Not slippery, unsteady, or uneven. Research tells us that we Seniors recover less easily from slips than those kids sixty-five and under do.

Be careful looking upward.

Avoid looking backward unless you can hold on to something. It may be better to turn all the way around.

Don't rush around. Be patient.

Carrying anything is potential trouble. Avoid if possible.

GETTING OUT OF BED

The only thing the experts can think of is that sometimes if we Seniors get up too fast, we may get dizzy. But did anyone have to tell us at our age to start the day slowly? Probably not!

TAKING A SHOWER OR BATH

Taking a bath. We Seniors also generally remember after a time to test the water temperature in the tub or shower before we get in. And if we take a shower with our glasses on, as I used to do, experts suggest we clean the glasses off if they steam up or get water specked.

It was probably not a good idea when younger, however I found that it was the one time all day when my glasses got really clean. It was a hangover from steadier times, and Nance figured I should give it up. So I did. This time, don't do as I did.

If there's nothing else to grab, you can *touch* the top pole above the tub of shower for balance.

Just touch—without putting any weight on it. A better solution is to have grab bars put in or get one of those handy snap on grips that I later describe in the part about travel away from home.

Soap is slippery. Because soap is so slippery, keep one hand free so you can grab on if you need to. Liquid soap dispensers are available that attach to shower stalls.

Drying off. A main problem is in covering your eyes. Either hold on or do one eye at a time.

DRESSING

Slipping pants on. Seniors know that if they have a balance problem, it helps to sit down or lean against a wall when putting on pants or slacks. Walls are good friends.

Walking around in our socks. If we Seniors walk around our homes in our stocking feet, our pants or slacks will drag down close to the floor and may trip us up. Socks always seem to work down and flop beyond the toes and when they do, they will trip us. And socks are also slippery.

One study found that walking barefoot reduced the stress and impact on the knees by 12 percent. It's why walking barefoot on the beach is so pleasant, and I do it around the house when I can. Slippers with a rubber soles are also advisable.

Untied shoelaces. If you step on an untied shoe lace with the other foot and then try to take a step, you are likely to fall. Take my word for it, I've tried it. Seniors are advised to find a place to sit down and tie them. Or let me suggest to inveigle someone to kneel at our feet and do it for us, like the prince did for Cinderella. An easier solution may be to get shoes with Velcro straps or a zipper.

Dressing sticks. We Seniors may also find one or more of these useful—a dressing stick (a rod with hook on the end) to pull on pants or socks, an elongated shoehorn, or a nab-grabber to safely extend our reach Nance uses one of our grabbers to get down clothes stuck in the chute, an added benefit.

Long sleeves. Probably all of us Seniors have had our sleeves catch on door handles as we go through or on railings at the tops of stairs or even on the tops of fancy dining room chairs. That's scary. About the only thing we can do is not to rush around and watch what we're doing. Or we can button them or wear short sleeves as I do.

Sitting. After an hour or so of sitting, stand, and if you are not dizzy, take a walk.

Wandering Around the House

Floor clutter. It gives many of us Seniors a fine feeling to toss unopened junk mail around our chair with the intention of looking at it someday. Or we may conveniently discard sections of the morning newspaper, a magazine, or even books onto empty floor spaces.

We may like to take our shoes off and to keep them handy or remove a sweater when it gets warm, drop it nearby, and think that we'll hang it up later. After a while, we may feel we've had enough from our heating pad but may want to use it again soon. Like the blanket that we've used to keep our legs warm or our cane, we'll just put them on the floor near our easy chair.

Just remember what our mothers said about picking up after ourselves, and, this time, there's a good reason for us unsteady Seniors finally to follow her advice. We can stumble or we can get hemmed in. Either one can result in a fall.

But sometimes it's not even our fault. Grandkids may leave their toys scattered around on the rug while they run off for lunch. So, sailor, beware.

Our pets. Love them, but watch out that you don't stumble over your Dundee or Mopsie or step on them. Other pet related obstacles are their chewy toys, water and food dishes, and their leashes. Have you ever tried to put a cat on a leash?

A study by the Centers for Disease Control covering the period 2001 to 2006 found that 235 persons every day show up in emergency rooms injured by pets. That comes to eighty-six thousand a year. Eighty-eight percent of the injuries were caused by dogs. Women were twice as likely to be injured then men. The most common injuries were to the arm and hand (27%), followed by the head and neck, and the leg and foot (24% each). Thankfully, only eleven percent involved the lower torso FYI.

Spills. Wipe up spills immediately. On second thought, get a Dundee, it's easier than stooping down, and you'll make a friend at the same time.

Turning on a low lying TV or VCR/DVD player. Use the TV remote rather than fiddling with the buttons on the set. And if the VCR or

DVD player is located down below the set, let someone else crawl down there and load in the movies.

Stairs. It's generally not a good idea to rush, especially when going down stairs. Steps that are only three or four inches high are a special pain.

As Don will explain, there is no safe method for falling down stairs, unless maybe you're a professional movie stunt man, and I hear some of them come out pretty battered.

When the heel lands on the edge of the step we stand a good chance of tilting forward and losing our balance. One way to prevent this is to angle our feet so most or all of each foot is fully on the stair tread.

However, the main thing is not to let your hands get too far from those friendly railings. Also, grip them with your thumb opposite your fingers for better support so that the hand does not slip off.

It often seems convenient to stack things on the bottom steps when we want to take them upstairs later. It's not the best idea we've ever had.

Take it from me, carrying anything on the stairs is—well, think about it first.

Going Outside

Stumbling over curbs. Researchers have drummed into our heads that we should check the height of curbs before stepping up or down. What they should also say is that we Seniors should look out especially for something we didn't expect, such as a two inch high curb or those slanted cutaways for bicycles.

Getting down icy stairs. If we Seniors feel we just have to go down icy stairs for the mail or the *Lansing State Wahoo* or whatever, we are told to grasp the railing with both hands and go up and down sideways, stepping on each stair with one foot and then the other.

On icy ground. The researchers advise us to inch our way forward or turn sideways and take small sidesteps, or if we are somehow caught out there in a really dangerous patch, we should just sit down and bump and slide ourselves forward on you know what.

Unexpected slippery spots. We are told we shouldn't let our guard down outside when walking on slanting or uneven surfaces. We know enough to be careful walking on wet leaves but sometimes over look the small leaves from trees like locusts and may not be aware what dry pine needles can do for us.

Wearing sunglasses. We know we should wear sunglasses when the glare from snow or sand or anything else may bother us. On the other hand, remember why they tell us to take them off when driving through a tunnel? You may get the same effect going inside the house with them on.

Shoulder bags. In bad weather especially using, a shoulder bag keeps our hands free.

Layering. In cold weather, the researchers suggest Seniors wear three layers of clothes and peel off layers if they get warm. The first layer can be tied around the waists, but what happens to the second layer is a subject that the experts don't address.

The inner layer should be synthetic, the middle layer wool, and the outer layer a water resistant jacket. Stay away from cotton shirts and socks in cold weather. They soak up sweat like a sponge and if we're damp; we Seniors are going to be cold.

The researchers say two light-weight pairs of socks or gloves are better than one heavy pair. And petroleum jelly on the face prevents chapping.

Padded underwear. If we have had multiple falls, it might be a good idea in winter weather to think about padded underwear to protect the hips. Or we could put on a heavy down jacket. Studies in Finland, which I'm told is a frosty place, found a reduction of 84 percent in hip fractures for those who wore hip pads.

Some wearers of the older hip protectors reported they got hot and uncomfortable, but it may be worth it for those at high risk. But light-weight protective pads have now been developed that can be worn next to the skin, and we can be sure someone will be happy to sell them to us unsteady Seniors. One brand has its shields sewn into the undergarment.

DRIVING OFF SOMEWHERE FOR A WILD DAY IN TOWN

Canes. Keep an extra one in the car.

Facing a car seat. When unsteady Seniors feel unsure about in getting or out of a car, the researchers say we'll find it helpful to follow the ladylike strategy. We get in sideways, our rear end in first, holding on where we can, but we don't let our weight down fully until we feel the seat on the back of our legs. This is a good idea elsewhere as well. Then we swing our legs around.

Getting out we reverse the process, but hold on to the door frame and look down to find out what kind of stuff we might be stepping out onto or into. This way even gentlemen can not only look ladylike but be in control, which all of us males like. Actually, they now sell swivel cushions that they claim makes getting in and out even easier.

Finding your theater seat. When unsteady Seniors arrive at an auditorium, they may find that their seats are five steps up, just off the center aisle, and not along a wall where those friendly railings hang out. Their best bet for is to hold on to the arm of a more stable friend. They like helping out. It gives them a sense of being useful.

Another danger situation is when it stops snowing, and we have to face one of those steep and sometimes long shallow steps with no railings in sight. These are doozies because we are mixing walking forward with shallow steps down.

It helps to keep a cane handy even if we have friends along. I've found we have to remind our sometimes forgetful pals who we may want to hang on to them when the performance is over. They may just charge out ahead and leave us stranded trying to keep our balance by grabbing on to the backs of seats or strangers. It's best to arrive at a movie before the lights go out. Getting there a little early means you may have to listen to endless advertisements about the local dentist and the refreshment stand. Then have to close our eyes and eat popcorn during all those slam-bang-crash previews of "coming attractions."

In restaurants. I take a cane when I go to crowded and unfamiliar restaurants where there may be steps with no railings. You don't always need it, but it helps to know it's there.

This is where people most often seem to forget canes. It's hard to find a place to put them without tripping up the waiter or a passing customer. I find it easiest to keep the cane between my legs, just as in a theater.

WHILE TRAVELING

Motels. We should be able to take for granted that all modern chains will have grab bars in their shower-tub combinations. Regrettably, this is not the case. In such an up-to-date community as Holland, Michigan, a motel of a national chain, otherwise very nice and modern, lacked those helpful and useful steadiers. If this is the case, join my campaign of telling the management about it on one of those suggestion cards they generally leave lying around.

Now available are handle grips with suction cups. The important part is that they have switches at each end that squeeze all the air out. They cost around fifteen dollars and really work on tile but less so on painted walls. They need only be touched for balance but will even support some weight.

Rubber bath mats. When traveling, especially abroad, many unsteady Seniors find it useful to take along a rubber bath mat, especially for those high bath tubs the English seem to admire so much.

Also, a night light may sometimes come in handy but only in the U.S. and Canada. Ours will blow out plugged into Europe's 250 volts.

Revolving doors. Avoid them when you can. They can be harder or easier to push than you expect, and someone is almost always coming along behind you who is in a hurry.

Public buildings and banks. They often have marble floors to show us taxpayers and depositors that our money is going to a noble cause. You may face a yellow triangular sign up that says, "Slippery when wet." Hold on to someone or something, or find a dry route.

Cyclists and skateboarders. Probably the best strategy is to stand still, hold on to something if you can, and hope for the best as they pass by.

PRECAUTIONS WHILE MOVING ABOUT
WHAT WAS THAT CHAPTER ALL ABOUT?

The goal is to avoid problems as we navigate. The experts have a variety of suggestions you can take or leave or maybe even laugh at. The general rules are to avoid the dark, check where you step for anything slippery, slanted, or unsteady, watch out when looking up or back, and don't rush around.

There were suggestions for handling problems we may face in getting out of bed, taking a shower or bath, dressing, wandering around the house, going outside, driving off somewhere for a wild day in town, and keeping balance in the midst of daily activities.

Chapter 12

The Unsteady Senior Reviews

Hazards around the Home

We know "the basic rule." Don't take foolish chances!

But do we always heed this advice?

So here are a few suggestions to fix things around the house to protect you from your own foolishness. Let your eyes glaze over, or just glide down the list and stop when you find something useful.

As with any list of suggestions on navigating, I sometimes feel a little silly mentioning the obvious or sometimes listing the wildly improbable hazard. Sort these out on our own. Pick out what's helpful to you. Someone thought they were hazards regardless what you or I think.

The General Rules

These are the ways to make things safer.

Check your home room by room. Brian Franklin, a certified athletic trainer at University Orthopedics in Atlanta and the MetLife Foundation, recommends that you consciously take a good look at your day-to-day surroundings to discover where danger spots might lurk.

Look around for things to get rid of. Check out things you may trip over or that can cause you to slip and anything that is as unsteady as you are. These could be rickety chairs or flimsy end tables, convenient to grab in an emergency, and get rid of throw rugs.

Look for stumble hazards. Take a look around your house at what you might stumble over, especially in the semidark. Rearrange for unobstructed and wide enough paths for you to navigate between hassocks, coffee tables, floor lamp cords, etc.

Good lighting is nonnegotiable. Lamps and light switches should be handy where you enter a room, so you don't have to grope around in the dark. Switches that glow in the dark are useful.

Now let's get specific about changes we might want to make.

Consumer Products That Injure

The National Safety Council tabulated the annual number of injuries from various products. These were serious enough to send people to emergency rooms.

Their figures include people of all ages, not just us unsteady Seniors. You may be astonished with what they found.

Omitted from this list were injuries from such obvious hazards as guns, saws, knives, ladders, scissors, ovens, and of course stairs. Stairs are not considered a consumer product.

You may have to puzzle a while to figure out how someone could hurt themselves on some of these. However, you might expect someone to fall out of bed or out of a rickety chair when it collapsed.

Kids swallowing coins happen, but you're on your own with household containers and packaging. Check out the following list.

The products are categorized by number of injuries sustained.

518,441	beds and bedding
306,523	chairs
223,260	household containers and packaging
145,936	sofas, divans, and davenports
121,094	footwear
107,052	tableware (excluding knives)
79,753	jewelry
64,216	toilets
42,811	televisions

The 23,000 to 40,000 injuries from highest to lowest were from pencils, pens, desk supplies, aquariums, pet products, refrigerators, coins, paper products, and sinks.

Still, I'm not sure how helpful this all is, but there it is. My hope is that you found it mildly interesting or amusing.

IN OUR BATHROOMS

This is where most of the serious falls that you read about in the newspapers happen. Winston Churchill slipped and fell there, though one always suspects a stimulant of choice may also have been involved.

Grab bars. Grab hand rails near the toilet and bath tub and in shower stalls are a must. Don't expect hot and cold fixtures or soap dishes, or the rail that holds the shower curtain to hold you up, though they may be *touched* to keep balance. If you put any weight on them, you are inviting a fall.

The screwed on rails are the best. But as already noted, you can now get hand rails that snap on to shower walls, and they really will hold your weight short of grabbing them as you fall. They work best on tile and not so well on painted walls.

The shower stall is damp. Mildew may grow under one of the discs of the snap on ones. If that happens, the fool thing will fall off. So check it if it seems a little loose, and scrub the disc and wipe it dry and clean.

Tub rails may be clamped on the side of the tub and held in place with a turn screw knob.

Tub Nonslip. If the tub doesn't have a built-in nonslip surface, put in a rubber mat or some of those nonslip cheery flower decals.

Carpeting the bathroom. Carpeting allows us to step out of the bathtub or shower stall with wet feet onto something other than slippery tile. If not carpeting, then put a rubber-backed bath mat near the tub or shower. It's marginally better than wet tile, I guess.

Night lights. They are a must in the bath room, between bed and bath room, and on dark stairways or in dark halls.

Raised toilet seat. Thoughtful manufacturers are now turning out toilets fourteen inches high for homes, hotels, and motels, intent on attracting only six-year-olds. Some Seniors have installed one of those eighteen-inch-high toilets or have installed a raised seat.

A padded shower chair. Those of us Seniors who have trouble getting out of the tub, even with grab bars, may get a padded shower chairand install a handheld shower hose.

Some may want a chair even if they have a walk-in shower.

Liquid soap dispensers. These attach to the shower wall. The ones I've seen screw on. All of us have had a bar of soap or shampoo bottle slip out of our hands. Picking up such slippery objects with hot water streaming down on us is a kind of neat trick.

Call-for-help buttons. They only work if the person called is also within the house, but that may be enough.

Bathroom door locks. Many locks allow someone to open them from the outside by inserting a nail in a slot on the outer knob. This is useful if you do have a fall, or you can just leave the door unlocked and hope for the best.

In Our Bedrooms

Bedroom lamps. You need a lamp and its light switch close to your bed, as well as an overhead light for when you come in.

Clothes hampers. It's not a good idea to scatter shoes and socks or clothing you take off as you undress to go to bed, especially where you may walk at night. You knew that but maybe you or your spouse does it anyhow. The same is true of the pile that you intend to put down the chute sometime later. Go to the trouble of using the hamper like mother always said.

Flashlights. Buy a flashlight to keep next to your bed and in a place where you can find it in the dark. Lately, one dark night, I learned this the hard way when I was reading in bed and the power went out.

It lasted for four hours. I spent an interesting ten minutes feeling around in the dark for the flashlight. You can now buy flashlights that are reenergized by pulling a cord, thus getting rid of worrying about rundown batteries. You can hardly have too many flashlights around the house.

Clocks. The best ones have large numerals that light up so you can read them without your glasses at night. Make sure the backup battery is in and charged. You may also get a light-up wrist watch.

Glasses at night. If you need glasses to see at night, put them in the same special place every day near the bed. They now have little felt-lined holders that stand up on a bedside table.

Monkey poles. This trapeze-like thing hangs from the ceiling. It is only for those who have really serious trouble getting out of bed. (Franklin Roosevelt pops up again.)

STAIRWAYS SHOULD GET OUR SPECIAL ATTENTION

The only fall that you can't break is a fall down a stairs.

Lighting stairwells. Switches at the top and bottom of Stairs are very handy, but if they aren't in already, it's too late for this. Maybe you can install a night light or one of those motion-detector lights that automatically turn on for a few minutes.

High-wattage lights. Put in high-wattage light bulbs on stairs as well as in hallways. Replace the hard to get at ones with the new florescent screw in bulbs that are supposed to last up to seven years. However, they seem to take twenty seconds or more to warm up to full strength.

Burned out light bulbs. When a bulb burns out, replace it. However, if it is on the ceiling, let someone else put it in.

Rounded hand rails. On staircases, especially the one to the basement, install rails on both sides and rubber stair treads or carpet. Rounded rails are easier to grab.

Keep stairs and halls clear. Don't stack things you want to take upstairs later on stairways or scatter galoshes or extra pairs of shoes around in the hall.

Thick carpeting on stairs. You may not think that thick carpeting on the stairs is a hazard, and I didn't either until I walked down such a set of stairs. The problems are that the surface area on the step is smaller and the edge is a little harder to see. We unsteady Seniors already have enough trouble with steep stairs.

It is easier to see the edge of the step if the carpeting is a solid color rather than a pattern. Regardless, hold on at all times.

Reflecting tape or paint. This is useful on the last step of a wood basement stairs or on the edges. Or use white or yellow paint.

THE OTHER ROOMS INSIDE OUR HOUSE

Flashlights. You can't have too many flashlights scattered around the house. With the pull-type or the self-contained, throwaway lights, we don't have to fiddle with batteries when they get dim. The very tiny ones are bright and fit easily in our pockets. They are great in emergencies, but they often get jarred, turn themselves on, and burn out. They are also useful to read restaurant menus in dim romantic settings.

Often times, I also carry a small magnifier and a tape measure too. That's why Nance says my pockets bulge.

Kitchen shelves. Keep frequently used kitchen items like dinner plates or platters on shelves within reach and not where you have to stoop or to stand on a stool to get to them. Anything on a high shelf needs to be near the edge to see it, and if it's heavy, getting it down can be tricky.

You can get long grabbers for light items on top shelves.

Waxed floors and throw rugs. Putting nonskid pads under the rugs won't help much, and it is better to avoid using them. Carpeting, anyway, is easier to take care of than waxed floors.

Basement doors. The actor David Niven lost his wife who, while playing a party game in someone else's home, opened a basement door in the dark and fell down the stairs.

In your own home, you can install a night light or motion-detector light. In other people's homes, take special care if for some reason, you need to open a closed door off the kitchen or dining room, especially if the light is dim.

The dining room table. Ones with four legs are usually steadier than the pedestal tables, which may tilt if you put your weight on them.

Easy chairs. Your favorite chairs should be high and have arms.

Fluorescent lights. They are said to last longer than ordinary bulbs and are said to be brighter.

Cordless Telephones You'll find it helpful to have a telephone near your favorite chair so you don't have to jump up and rush to the phone before it stops ringing. Cordless phones that can be lifted out of the holder is one option, but cell phones are almost a must for unsteady Seniors.

You may prefer to use an answering machine to screen your calls. Unfortunately, you will miss out from responding to those plastic siding salesmen and never-heard-of-before charities, if you like that sort of thing.

Uneven floors. Repair buckling or other uneven spots on floors. Seems silly to say, but we've had friends who ignored them for years. They got used to them; however, their visitors didn't.

Raised thresholds. Enough said.

Electrical cords. Hide all of them including computer cords. Use a twisty tie to shorten cords.

Rugs under a heavy center table. They bunch up around the edges as if by magic. My carpet store friend told me that the fix was to move the coffee table off the rug, straighten it out, and then drag or push the table back. Somehow, I had hoped for a different answer.

Corners of rugs can also be treacherous when they curl up.

Drapes. Even long drapes or table cloths that lap out onto the floor or close to it can trip us up. Some say they look sloppy anyhow. Others say they're artistic.

No-bend Dustpans. A dustpan with a broom handle attached, they are very handy, especially if you shatter a glass.

Laundry. Have a stool near the dryer if bending is a problem. Carry laundry up or down steps in a bag that you can hold in one hand, so say the experts.

Newspapers and mail. Ask the carrier to put newspapers in the same, easily accessible place, and good luck. They may need a generously tip at Christmas as an incentive to get exactly what you want.

Have your mailbox near the door if possible, especially if you live where it snows.

Doors. If you have trouble opening doors, have lever-type handles installed. If it's a big problem, and you don't care about cost, check out electronic door openers.

AND OUTSIDE OUR HOMES

Motion-detector lights. Install motion-detector lights for outside illumination. They are useful and cheap and will stay lit for several minutes after being activated.

Cracked sidewalks. Get the city to repair sidewalks, especially where tree roots push them up, and, again, good luck.

Garden paths. You can use spray-on products to kill slippery moss or grass that grow over the stones. However, beach grass at our cottage seems to thrive on the stuff.

Florescent paint. Dabble it around the front door keyhole if that's the way you come in at night. Others suggest you also may want to paint the last step of your front porch steps with nonslip white or yellow paint.

Or then again, you may not want to light up the neighborhood this way.

AN UNRELATED THOUGHT

Restaurants: Some now have booths that hold up the table top without legs that you have to crawl over and around. It might be a good idea to reward such places with our patronage.

HAZARDS AROUND THE HOME
WHAT WAS THAT CHAPTER ALL ABOUT?

Check your home room by room. Look around for things to get rid of. Look for stumble hazards. Good lighting is nonnegotiable. We then tour the house from bedroom and bathroom and outside looking for what might trip us up.

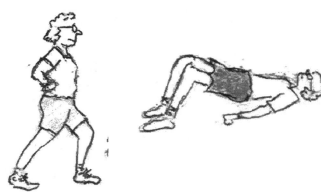

Chapter 13

A Final Note From the Unsteady Senior

The deadly killer for us grown-ups is *sloth*! For unsteady Seniors, it heads the lineup of those Seven Deadly Sins. We can deal with greed and lust and the other four some other time.

Let's go over it one more time. If we become inactive and stop doing things, we slowly and gradually begin to fall apart, piece by piece, limb by limb, toenail by toenail, molecule by molecule.

Depression then walks in upon the scene. We need medication, the kind of doses that add to the profits of those poor poverty-stricken pill makers. The next step for us is, pretty soon, we are the featured performer in a spectacular fall.

And consider how activity benefits our brains and personalities. Try it. Ask your spouse, or a friend, if you don't seem more intelligent and scintillating lately.

Actually, scientists aren't kidding. They think there's something to this. Henriette van Praag of the Salk Institute for Biological Studies in San Diego found new neurons being formed in the brains of mice that were put on running wheels. Other studies showed that Seniors who are active score better on mental tests. Oh boy!

Of Course There Are Limits

Sooner or later, we all come across a newspaper article about a Senior aged eighty-three trudging down the Appalachian Trail or on a predawn jaunt up the Andes mountains. If that's your thing, go for it.

But there are other alternatives for the rest of us that still result in an active and satisfying life.

A FINAL TIP

This handbook is an action book. Don't just read through to the end and put it down. Refer to it as you exercise. As I've already noted, I can't count the times I've gone back and looked at the details in some of Don's chapters or even my own chapters. We forget, or maybe we didn't read it carefully enough the first time. Go back and refer!

WHAT YOU CAN ACCOMPLISH

If you do half of what Don and I recommend and keep at it, it will help with your unsteadiness and reduce the probabilities that you will fall. The researchers say so, the medical profession says so, and Don and I say so. How much you improve depends on when you start and how faithfully you keep at it.

Doing those muscle twitches though still eludes me. I'm saving them for my nineties.

That's it. Cheers!

PART TWO

What an Experienced Physical Therapist Says about Balance for Unsteady Seniors

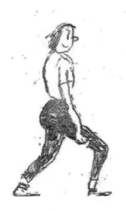
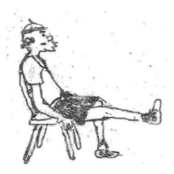

Chapter 14

The Mechanisms of Balance

Balance Disorders: Life-Altering Conditions

They begin with, compensatory maneuvers ultimately progress to a point of dependency in even the basic elements of living. The fear of falling is in itself self-limiting, but actual falls frequently result in debilitating fractures, loss of independence, social withdrawal, and depression.

Should this be the accepted progression for Seniors or are there options and opportunities to reverse this malady?

Reversing the decline. You are embarking on a program to reverse this decline: to return to walking more normally, to allow you to put on pants while holding on or sitting, and perhaps to get the mail out of the box without losing your balance.

It is imperative that you understand the mechanisms of balance. Only then will you be able to relate to exercises specific to your particular problems.

No one was born with balance skills. They were developed over time in conjunction with other physiological changes. Your first attempts at sitting and standing were met with failure, but you eventually succeeded. Yet, over the years, generalized strength and flexibility gradually regressed, but it was the balance issues that told us we have a problem!

However, balance is a motor skill that can improve with practice and that means at any age. The logical progression of an exercise program is to begin with the simple and then to advance to the complex.

Hopefully, the following concepts will give you the understanding of balance principles needed to pursue these exercises logically and purposefully.

MECHANISM 1
BALANCE REQUIRES THE COOPERATION OF MANY SYSTEMS

Physical problems such as back and neck ailments, osteoarthritis, osteoporosis, sprains, and/or pains in the weight-bearing joints can result in altered body mechanics leading to balance problems.

These have to be taken care of, to the extent possible, before beginning an exercise program. Unless we correct that which is treatable, our exercise program may be counterproductive and may even do harm. So before you begin, consult your physician.

Conditions such as arthritis, osteoporosis, and mild sciatica may all benefit from exercise. But for these, and others, see your physician before you begin. Actually, this advice is good for all unsteady Seniors. Your physician knows a good deal about your physical condition and can offer useful suggestions.

MECHANISM 2
PROPER POSTURE: HUMANS ARE TOP HEAVY

The human frame is essentially unstable. Two-thirds of our body mass is located in the upper two-thirds of our height. Now, if we were Weeble Wobbles, we would teeter and not fall, but we are not, and so we are in danger of falling.

A recovery program must begin by emphasizing proper posture.

The head is the control center for regulating the sensory input for balance. During the aging process, the head position seems to shift forward. Since the head serves as the reference source for upright posture, the difference between standing and falling is often in how we position our head. For this reason, conscious awareness of the head position is imperative whenever we sit, walk, or exercise.

MECHANISM 3
MAINTAINING SUFFICIENT FLEXIBILITY

This allows us to gain maximum benefit from exercising. Stretches that increase your range of motion are especially important for the arthritic and the sedentary. They are also useful for everyone for getting rid of morning stiffness and for warming up before exercising or cooling down afterward.

MECHANISM 4
STRENGTHENING MUSCLES

My son was born with a club foot and did not develop the strength sufficient for him to balance on that leg. Through karate, he was able to achieve seemingly impossible feats of balance through a well-orchestrated program of flexibility, strengthening, and balance activities.

As we age, Seniors lose muscle strength to the extent that instability becomes an issue. Just as the case with my son, strong legs, ankle muscles, and core muscles will help keep us unsteady Seniors from falling if we should begin to lose our balance.

MECHANISM 5
DEVELOPMENT OF STATIC BALANCE
AND POSTURAL REFLEXES

Many of the balance exercises require us unsteady Seniors to stand upright without moving our feet or arms. One example is doing the stork (standing on one leg without holding on). They are part of increasing our muscle memory.

As we become more proficient at this, we may assume that we have also achieved enhanced functional balance, that is balance as we move about, but this may not be the case.

Rehabilitation of our postural reflexes is equally, if not more, important. Balance exercises involving movement have to be introduced to help develop these reflexes. This includes such exercises such as walking a line heel to toe.

Mechanism 6
The Value of Light Touching

The final mechanism of balance involves the role that light touch plays in sustaining balance when walking or standing still. We may incorrectly assume that the use of a cane is unnecessary once we develop mule strength sufficient for stability. In reality, even the very light touch of a cane provides a source of sensory information required to prevent us losing balance.

Light touch means using a cane for orientation, not support. You will also find light touching of walls may also be helpful. Walls are good friends.

What Was That Chapter All About?

Six mechanisms are used to reverse the decline in balance:

>correcting physical problems to the extent possible
>maintaining posture principles
>enhancing flexibility
>strengthening muscles
>developing postural reflexes
>appreciating the value of light touching

Chapter 15

WHO SHOULD STOP READING
RIGHT NOW AND WHY?

Some of you already suspect that an exercise program is long overdue. Still you will need to check with your physician to see if it is right for you.

Here are some of the individuals who especially must check with their physicians before beginning.

The sedentary. You have been largely sedentary for years, maybe decades. You get out of breath climbing a flight of stairs. It takes a week to recover after mowing the lawn, even on a rider. Or you never get short of breath because you never do anything. Get an idea of what kind of exercise you may be considering, and take the program and your ideas with you on your doctor's visit.

The seriously overweight. Obesity cannot be overcome solely by exercise. Extreme caution must be observed since the heart and other body organs are doing all they can just to adapt to excessive weight. Get involved with an organized weight-loss program overseen by a physician and one with accountability as a motivator.

Those with major disabilities. Individuals affected with major medical conditions such as heart disease, diabetes, severe asthma, high blood pressure, and others are among those for whom exercise can have the greatest benefits or the gravest results. Extreme caution should be taken before undertaking even a mild exercise program and always with physician involvement.

Those who need hip or knee replacements or have been diagnosed with spinal stenosis. When pain inhibits your daily activities and persists even at rest, it's not the time to take on an exercise program.

Seniors who have been advised and cleared to have surgery to address problems like worn out hips, knees, etc., would be better off waiting until after their procedures to pursue balance exercises. Follow your orthopedist's advice with the pursuance of an exercise program being a post-op goal. Meanwhile, as Charlie says, "no refunds," you will need this handbook later.

If surgery is an option in the next year or two, get started now on an exercise program.

The light-headed. Don't take light-headedness lightly. It may be serious. If you are subject to frequent fainting spells or light-headedness, you must get it checked out now before reading another word.

Seniors who occasionally feel faint when looking up, when rolling over in bed, or when getting up too quickly from a bed or a chair may be suffering from a temporary decreased blood supply to the brain. The symptoms usually resolve quickly, but it is important for you to remain seated or to lie down until they do. If you try to "walk it off," you may fall.

If you want to do something to make it pass, try tightening your fists and arms, crossing your legs at the ankles, and bending them tightly, raising your arms over your head, contracting your abdominal muscles, or clasping your hands, entangling your fingers, and pulling the arms apart. *Do not hold your breath!*

Other causes of occasional light-headedness include pain, fatigue, anxiety, negative effects of medication, and the lack of food (low blood sugar).

Now that you have a list to choose from, pick out the culprit, and then do something about it.

In addition, always stand up slowly and look straight ahead.

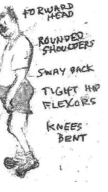

Those with stooped posture. Where the head goes, so goes the body. This is as true in gymnastics and diving as it is with someone who demonstrates a pronounced rounded back and forward head posture; such is typical in advanced osteoporosis. This is not an exclusive Senior condition but one that many Seniors have.

My advice is to see your physician who will determine if you are a candidate for a physical therapy assessment and customized exercise program. Only then will you be able to discern which of the exercises contained in this book may be helpful. Personal trainers familiar with osteoporosis may be another option.

The Mayo Clinic did a study of Seniors with osteoporosis using a device called a weighted kypho-orthosis (WKO). The participants exercised for four weeks while wearing the WKO harnessed to their backs, just below the shoulder blades. The researchers found significant improvement in balance, gait, and back strength as well as a reduction of pain.

Cancer patients. There may be a Senior out there having both impaired balance and cancer. The only reason you should stop reading right now is to get medical permission to exercise.

I once taught the exercise section on the "I Can Cope" cancer series. This consisted of presentations by various disciplines on management techniques for cancer patients in all phases of treatment. The value of exercise as part of cancer care was at that time under emphasized and rarely pursued.

The lazy. If you are among the few who are too lazy to get more involved in the life around you, stop reading right now. Instead, buy a motivational publication. The only thing that laziness promotes is more laziness. However, if you are the ultimate lazy, you won't even want to put out the energy to turn the pages of any book. On the other hand, if you have read this far, there is hope. See your physician and get started!

The very frail. Ten to fifteen percent of Seniors are in this category as a result of illness, malnutrition, being sedentary, or a combination of all these factors. Severe frailness is a chronic and progressive condition not easily reversed, especially by a self-help text like this.

The underlying pathology must be stabilized, and the nutritional component needs to be addressed to assure that there is adequate fuel to run both the bodily functions plus the added demands from exercising. You need help and begin by seeing your doctor.

THOSE HAVING MINOR COMPLAINTS

Impaired balance is often accompanied by other ailments such as arthritis, mild to moderate osteoporosis, and mild sciatica. For those Seniors, researchers have good news.

Exercise for those with these conditions can result in improvement in both strength and balance, so hang in there. Both the *Journal of Neurophysiology and Otology and Neurology* in 2004 stated that no matter what the cause for loss of balance, exercise can diminish the problem and reduce the risk of a fall.

Arthritis. In their June 27, 2005 roundup of information on arthritis, the *U.S. News and World Report* stated that doctors are "recognizing that managing arthritis often can be done by physical therapy rather than drugs." The Arthritis Foundation sponsors a program for arthritics, "People with Arthritis Can Exercise" (PACE).

Osteoporosis. The Cleveland Clinic recommends strengthening exercises to "stem bone loss" for those with osteoporosis. This will result in reducing the risk of fracture from brittle bones.

Sciatica. This disease is a syndrome characterized by pain radiating from the back into the buttocks and into the lower extremity. The term sciatica is also used to refer to pain anywhere along the course of the sciatic nerve (Dorland's Illustrated Medical Dictionary). The causes of sciatica vary widely from a minor malalignment to severe, secondary to disc pathology. Symptoms often resolve within months and up to a year even without treatment. The problem is that sciatica left untreated may needlessly get worse, making it very difficult to do any type of physical activity, let alone exercise.

Once cleared by your physician and therapy begins, insist on a home exercise program specific to your condition. That way you will be better able to do the exercises in this book without aggravating the sciatic symptoms.

AND FOR THE REST

It is good that some recognize they have a serious medical problem and want to do something about it because exercising in the presence of an undiagnosed, underlying medical problem could have undesirable results.

But it's not enough for others to say. "I keep losing my balance. But if I do what this handbook advises, I won't have to go see my doctor." Or "I've always wanted to exercise; maybe now is the time since I have this handbook." "I've put on fifty pounds over the past ten years. It's about time to work out!"

Checking with your doctor. So what's the big deal? We are Seniors and should have gotten over physician phobia long ago.

If your intent is to bypass your physician's input, then stop reading right now. Regardless of your perceived fitness level, check with your physician to be sure than an exercise program is right for you.

What should you ask your physician? Be prepared to ask specific questions that require specific answers. A general question like "Should I exercise?" will induce an equally vague response. Have a good idea as to what kinds of exercises you have in mind.

Have a checklist of what you want to know. Write down your physician's comments. Are there any activities you shouldn't do? Also, get a copy of your vitals: weight, pulse, blood pressure, temperature, and heart rate.

If your physician does specific balance tests, make note of both the techniques used and the results. Ask about precautions specific to your condition. If you are still not sure where to go for your rehab, ask. All things considered, why wouldn't you want to see your doctor?

THE REST OF THE STORY

For an exercise program to be effective, it takes time and effort. As Seniors, we should have all the time in the world, but in reality we need to make time. If you are unwilling to dedicate a specific time each day to an exercise program, then stop reading right now.

Exercising to achieve fitness or to minimize disability requires a long-term commitment. This is not a two-credit physical education course. If you are not motivated to accept this challenge, then stop reading right now.

WHAT WAS THAT CHAPTER ALL ABOUT?

Seniors who have been especially sedentary, have a heart condition, are in respiratory distress, have uncontrolled blood pressure (high or low), experience frequent fainting spells, or have other debilitating conditions need to consult their doctors before getting into an exercise program.

Seniors who have been advised and cleared to have surgery to address problems like worn out hips, knees, etc., would be better off waiting until after their procedure to pursue balance exercises. If surgery is an option in the next year or two, get started now.

Seniors looking for an excuse not to exercise, being very, very frail is a good one because an exercise program is unlikely to help. However, if your medical conditions include arthritis, osteoporosis or sciatica, researchers say, "No excuse—exercise is *okay*."

All Seniors, in fact, should check with their physician before embarking on an exercise program.

Chapter 16

HOW BALANCE-CHALLENGED ARE YOU?

If you are planning on doing a "balance makeover," it makes sense to track your own progress from beginning to end. Discouragement often comes from our inability to see progress that others may be admiring. By conducting self tests on a regular basis, perhaps every other month, objective feedback is available in the comfort of your own home.

Your balance problems may be secondary to a sudden onset of a vestibular disturbance or to a gradual and progressive tendency to lose your balance and in the inability to regain it. Read on and you should be able to tell the difference between these conditions as well as what to do about it.

VESTIBULAR DISORDERS

The word "vestibular" refers to the inner ear. The vestibular system's primary function is in the area of balance. It provides the input about the body's movement and orientation. The Vestibular Disorders Association lists eighteen specific disorders, but only one will be addressed here—"Benign Paroxysmal Positional Vertigo" or in short "vertigo."

Vertigo. Vertigo is an illusion of movement. Sometimes just with a slight turn of the head, you experience the sensation that the world around you is revolving, or the external world is standing still and you are revolving. Nausea usually accompanies the spinning sensation.

These sensations can last from seconds to minutes and usually go away by lying still. However, they will reappear with another change in position.

Vertigo may result from diseases to the inner ear or possibly due to disturbances of the vestibular centers. Regardless of the cause, vertigo requires medical attention and professional treatment.

It is common for Seniors to compensate for their vestibular disorders by relying on visual cues. If you suspect you are doing this, try the following test.

A test for vertigo. Stand next to something that you can grab hold of and recruit someone to stand beside you. Close your eyes and let go. Can you hold your position for ten seconds? If you can do this, it means that you don't require your eyes for cues. If you fail to hold the position with your eyes closed, your problem may likely be vestibular. However, if you pass this test but still have balance problems, then you are ready to move on.

THE SOMATOSENSORY SYSTEM

There are sensors in our feet that send messages to the brain relaying information relative to their position. When operating normally, this somatosensory system permits us to correct positions that may lead us to lose our balance.

Conditioning exercises will be presented for this system to enhance better interpretations of incorrect positions and to instill responses that both restore and maintain balance.

STRENGTH TRAINING FOR MUSCLES THAT AID BALANCE

Another phase of training involves physical ability to restore and to maintain balance. This may involve your core strength and/ or your ankles and leg muscles or flexibility. Impaired balance and falling often results from the body's inability to correct something the somatosensory system already told the brain that the body needed to address.

Documenting Balance Measures

It is a good idea to occasionally test your balance. These tests can be simple or complex, but, to be reliable, they must be able to be accurately reproduced in order to come to any conclusions regarding balance changes. Even a slight change in technique, like the width of your stance, can give misleading findings.

When choosing one or more balance tests, document each and every variable such as follows:

> width of stance
> floor covering: carpet, hardwood, etc.
> visual distractions: looking out the window or at an interior wall
> audio distractions or quiet
> time of day
> type of footwear or bare feet
> before or after a meal
> amount of clothing you are wearing
> the amount of light in the room

Types of Balance

We begin testing three categories of balance: the static, the functional, and the force-response.

Static tests assess balance while standing or sitting without movement. Functional assessments determine your state of balance while you are doing something like walking, turning, bending, etc. The third type gives an indication on how you are able to respond to external forces in regaining your balance.

For example, you are outside with a fairly strong wind blowing. Will you remain upright? You are attending your fiftieth-year class reunion, and someone slaps you on the back. Will this put you on the floor, or will you respond with "Glad to see you, old man!"

It is obvious that some of these tests are designed to be performed by professionals and some on your own. As a cautionary warning, if you perceive that you may be balance impaired, have someone close by to assist you if necessary.

STATIC BALANCE TESTS

Romberg's Test. Stand on both feet in front of a perpendicular reference point such as a window frame or a wall with your eyes open for one minute. Repeat for one minute with your eyes closed. Have a spotter observe and record if you sway in relation to the reference point.

The Collins Test. Researcher, Dr. Jim Collins, is experimenting with a low-cost balance assessment technique. He has Seniors stand in place for a period of time and measures all the movements that take place. If you choose to do this, be consistent with the testing variables previously mentioned. Collins suggests that results from this technique may be as good as the more-complicated methods requiring special equipment.

The Stork Test. Stand on one foot bending the opposite leg's hip and knee so the toe/foot is held just above the floor surface. Arms may be held out to the side but keep your eyes open. Count to fifteen without holding on. Can you make thirty? Try waving your arms and see how much you wobble. Now try the stork with the other foot. Are you better on one than the other?

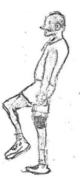

Keep in mind that walking is merely balancing on one foot then the other. Balance-challenged Seniors compensate for their inability to do so by shuffling, by walking with their legs far apart, or by holding on to something or someone.

FUNCTIONAL BALANCE TESTING

When you are engaged in everyday activities, are you putting yourself at risk of losing your balance and possibly falling? If so, read on.

Do you lose your balance as you bend over to pick up something or to tie your shoes? What about putting on or taking off a sweater or a polo shirt? Are just standing and walking challenges?

Low blood pressure. Rising quickly from a sitting or lying down position can result in a light-headed or head-swimming sensation. This is not vertigo. Although you may be at risk of losing your balance, the underlying problem is orthostatic hypotension or low blood pressure.

Seniors are particularly vulnerable due to cardiovascular disorders or naturally have low blood pressure. See your doctor to assess your risk. Blood pressure testing devices are also easy to use in your own home. As a reminder, a sudden onset of dizziness may be an early warning sign of an impending stroke or a symptom of vertigo.

The Drunk Test. My physical therapy department participated in the SEE program. This Summer Exploratory Experience was an opportunity for soon-to-be-seniors in high school to spend one week each in six different hospital departments, thus promoting interest in health care careers. Christal was one of these seniors who chose to observe what goes on in physical therapy.

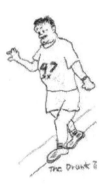

The Drunk?

Later on that summer, Christal also had the opportunity to be a "ride-along" with a patrol car officer. The officer spotted what appeared to be a staggering drunk making his way along a sidewalk. The drunk was being confronted when Christal spoke up, "He's not drunk; he has a neurologic condition. I saw him in therapy, and he always walks that way." The man was glad to see her!

Years later, Christal became a physical therapist. Seniors may wonder what would happen if a police officer stopped their car and demanded they walk a straight line. Cold, sober, they might end up you know where.

Find a straight line about ten feet long. It can be a crack where tiles are laid in a kitchen or in the mall, or you can put a string down on the carpet. Walk along it heel to toe, having your right foot always coming down on the line. Now do this with your left foot always hitting the line. Do you sway off the line more on one side than the other, or do you need to work on both directions?

Times Up-and-Go. Mark a spot ten feet ahead of an arm chair. Recruit a helper who will time your effort with a stopwatch. Sit down with your back touching the backrest. On "go," stand up walk to the spot at a normal pace, turn around, walk to the chair, and sit. A time of eight to ten seconds is normal; eleven to nineteen seconds indicates moderate risk of falling; twenty or more seconds signals a high risk.

FORCE-RESPONSE BALANCE TESTS

Professionals should supervise these tests because of the complex nature of the test, the safety factors, and because of their ability to accurately interpret the results.

Sitting. The Senior sits on a low table with feet touching the floor. The physical therapist pushes the Senior from the front, back, left, and right in no particular order or number of times. The ability of the Senior to maintain or to regain balance is assessed.

Standing. The same testing technique used in the sitting position is repeated with the Senior standing. The force-response tests will reveal strength deficiencies better than the other balance tests. The results will also help the therapist plan a rehabilitation program accordingly.

WHAT WAS THAT CHAPTER ALL ABOUT?

This section is all about balance assessment. It is not your responsibility to self-diagnose but rather to recognize that you may have a problem and then to find out what to do about it. The purposes of the self tests are to objectify balance deficiencies and to monitor subsequent changes.

You must decide on what direction to go in the rehab process. What to do may include attending physical therapy or exercising at a health club or at home.

Knowing these options is also useful when seeking physician input. Many patients are uninformed as to their health care options before seeing their doctor.

Chapter 17

Attending Physical Therapy

How Do I Get Physical Therapy?

Most states have direct access, meaning you can call the Physical Therapy Department to schedule an appointment. The rest of the states require a physician's referral for physical therapy. Regardless, you must have a medical need. It is not sufficient to just want a preventative or maintenance program.

Who Pays For It?

Providing there is medical need, insurance companies and Medicare will cover the expenses for a specific period of time, providing improvement can be documented. There may be out-of-pocket expenses in the way of copays and/or deductibles. It is always a good idea to check your policy for details.

What Should I Expect?

You will receive an evaluation by a physical therapist. This will include consideration of your history, any test results (x-rays, etc.), and physical findings by the therapist. A rehabilitation program will be customized specific to your needs. The treatment plan will be modified as changes occur. You will be expected to be compliant in your attendance as well as with the home program the physical therapist recommends for you. You will also have a professional available to answer your questions.

EQUIPMENT

Unresolved pain and other deterrents to exercising can be addressed by equipment specific to physical therapy departments. Exercise equipment will vary greatly from one facility to the other.

Treadmill and stationary bikes. These are two pieces of equipment that Seniors with balance problems will find most useful. Treadmills are bulky but do have handrails on which to hold on while walking. Stationary and recumbent bikes can be used for individuals who are unable to walk on treadmills. Both treadmills and stationary bikes are excellent for warm-ups and aerobic conditioning.

Weight machines. They have an advantage over free weights because they don't require the degree of conditioning that free weights do. The disadvantage is that the stronger extremity can compensate for the weaker one.

A MAINTENANCE PROGRAM

Check with your physical therapist to see if the clinic offers a maintenance program. For a nominal fee this permits you to return and use the facilities' exercise equipment.

A home program. A home program should be initiated early in the therapy series. This will permit modifications and clarifications if needed. Your supplemental home program will be refined to address your short—and long-term needs.

Some of the pieces of equipment used in physical therapy are not so expensive or complex that a Senior couldn't buy or make them for home use. Try them out first and figure out how long you may need to do the exercise before buying or building.

Elastic band. Elastic bands are about four inches wide. Elastic tubing is used in a similar way as the bands. They come in colors that vary according to the resistance they provide. Tension can also change according to how much stretch you put on the bands of any color.

Advantages include the following: They are lightweight and portable, like taking them on vacation. They are three-dimensional, meaning you can get resistance in any direction depending on where you attach it. You can simulate functional activities like reaching upward or recreational sports like a golf or tennis swing. As you gain strength, you can move up to a stronger band.

The disadvantages are that you may get accidently snapped; they do wear out in time; and your grandchildren may run off with them.

Exercise balls (also called Swiss balls, therapeutic balls or physioballs). These are large, somewhat-spongy plastic/vinyl balls with smooth or textured surfaces. Textured ball covers provide a grip and are bouncier and softer but have lower weight ratings.

These balls are one of the more dynamic yet gentlest method for improving balance and/or strength. Pilates has expanded its scope to include the use of Swiss balls. Physical therapy clinics have used them for years, and you will also find them in most health clubs. I have also seen them on cruise ships.

My advice is to be professionally trained in their use and to have a program designed to meet your individual needs. If this training comes through your physical therapist, you will be advised whether or not this is a good home exercise. If indicated, you will need to know what size ball, where to buy one, and what to do on it.

For around fifty dollars, you can purchase one. They are durable, but if one is punctured, never try to fix it. When sitting on one, your knees should be at right angles. A fifty-five-centimeter ball will fit someone 5'4" a sixty-five-centimeter ball will work for someone 5'11".

WHAT WAS THAT CHAPTER ALL ABOUT?

Physical therapists are professionals trained in dealing with balance-impaired individuals of all ages. Not only will you have a program specifically designed to meet your needs, but you will also have the opportunity to try out specific pieces of equipment. Your supplemental home program will be implemented into your primary and long-term exercise plan. This therapist may also end up being a resource person later on in life. Isn't that right, Charlie?

Chapter 18

Exercising at Health Clubs

There are some facilities that offer Senior discount memberships but restrict the hours, which may or may not be the best for you.

What Can Fitness Centers Offer?

1. 24-hour gym access
2. individual nutritional analysis
3. diet and weight loss programs
4. steam rooms and/or whirlpool baths
5. swimming pools
6. tanning
7. tennis, racket ball, and basketball courts
8. motivation, guidance, encouragement, and socialization
9. Senior discounts, perhaps if you ask for one
10. personal trainers

An Overview of the Equipment

Walk into any health club, and you will be dazzled by a landscape of sleek weight-lifting machines. These facilities are in the exercise business, and profits are based upon how many people can be accommodated. Thus, they have many "work stations."

Their machines are expensive, durable, and, once you learn what to do, user friendly. However, it would be difficult to buy one or more of these machines for home use.

On the other hand, you may have the opportunity to see how you and your body react to specific types of exercises like the stationary bikes and treadmills addressed earlier. Two additional ones are rowing machines and elliptical motion trainers.

Rowing machines. These are designed to build strength and endurance in the arms, shoulders, legs, and in the back, hips, knees, and ankles. Since the exercise is performed while sitting, incorporating alternate flexion and extension movements in the back, hips, and legs, those individuals with tight hamstrings, back inflexibility, or existing back problems should think twice before getting on one and only after seeking professional advice.

Elliptical trainers. Elliptical trainers mimic the body's natural movement. Foot plates travel around an axis in an elliptical pattern, and handles move back and forth. The differential advantage of this device is that it is an effective cardiovascular machine with significantly reduced impacts on the joints.

PERSONAL TRAINERS

Health club staff members are all knowledgeable in the physiology of exercise, how to operate their machines, and in the planning of workout routines. The amount of their education can differ widely. Beware of any medical advice, but heed their warnings should they suspect compromising health issues.

Personal trainers, on the other hand, may be well worth the extra expense. They should have a higher degree of exercise education than you plus a wealth of experience. Hiring one for a few sessions is a good way to get started.

COMMUNITY RESOURCES

1. Check the Yellow Pages under exercise to find health clubs.
2. Universities may open up their fitness facilities to the public. Seniors may get special rates.
3. Senior centers have exercise rooms.

4. Many YMCAs have gyms and/or swimming pools.
5. Schools may have public swims or aquatic programs for special needs like arthritis.
6. Even motels/hotels have equipment rooms that may be open to the public; just ask.

The Silver Sneaker Program. Free memberships for Seniors at selected health clubs are available through a program called Silver Sneakers. It works through some Medicare plans. To find out if you are eligible, contact www.silversneakers.com or call 1-800-295-4993.

WHAT WAS THAT CHAPTER ALL ABOUT?

There are two things you need to do before considering a fitness center. First, get medical clearance from your physician. Second, get insights if personal trainers are not available. It is perfectly acceptable to work on balance at home while enhancing your fitness levels in a gym.

Chapter 19

Exercising at Home

Being compliant with your home exercise program designed by a physical therapist is mandatory, but exercising on your own at home is optional.

If you opt out of the health club scene, you have some serious decisions to make. The second phase of your rehabilitation is the strengthening of your extremity and core muscles and the conditioning of your cardiovascular system. It makes sense to develop an effective exercise program in your home since you will be doing this for years to come.

A Home Exercise Program

You may be a Senior with a balance problem and have sought out professional assistance. You have been given a home exercise program; but now what? Follow the program to the letter, even if this means doing it three times a day. You will be reconditioning both your mind and body and this takes time and effort. This is phase one.

Exercising at home has advantages. You can dress as you wish, and makeup is optional. Drinks and emergency snacks are nearby. You will save on membership fees and on gas. There will be far less commotion in your home, and you can exercise at times convenient to you.

Disadvantages are that you are limited in your exercise option. Modifications in your program are up to you. Compliance may also be a major drawback. I have heard many people say that they will do something that they pay for but not if they have to do everything on their own.

Specific exercises that can be done at home will be addressed in subsequent chapters.

AN EXERCISE AREA

Designate a special area in your home exclusively for exercise. A spare room that you could fancy up is ideal if it can be cleared out. It's not safe to work out in a cluttered area. A suggestion is to put any dumbbells you have near the mirror so you don't stumble over them. Mirrors on at least one wall come in handy to check your posture and form.

Unfinished basements are my least favorite areas. They're not finished for a good reason; you don't go there. You want an exercise room that's inviting and one that "triggers the emotions."

Floor surfaces. Carpets with a short-napped and a quality pad will provide shock absorption for your feet and joints. Exercise mats come in various sizes and thicknesses. Choose one that fits your workout type. Carpet remnants are relatively inexpensive and may be ideal to put on concrete floors.

Buying equipment. Don't buy any piece of equipment until you have tried it. Every piece of equipment out there is marketed as the best in whatever the promoter promotes.

In reality, they are user specific. What works for me may not for you. What is ideal for the mister may be wrong for the mistress. What's on sale in the sporting goods department may be even a better buy at a garage sale next summer. A good deal is not a good reason to buy something.

I had several pieces of exercise equipment donated to my therapy clinic because the person who bought them was worse after using them.

Ask yourself these questions before buying equipment.

Do I know which parts of my anatomy need exercise?
Does this piece of equipment target these areas?
Considering all things, is this safe for me to use?

Can I afford it?
Do I have room for this piece of equipment?
Will I use it?

WHAT WAS THAT CHAPTER ALL ABOUT?

Exercising at home is optional. You need to find a bright and airy room to exercise in, preferably not in an unfinished basement. Think carefully before buying expensive equipment.

Chapter 20

Preparation for Exercising

Consider exercising with the same mind-set as you would have taking a road trip to parts unknown. AAA could provide you with a "Trip Tick," and you would get your vehicle checked out. Footwear and clothing options may require some thought as well. Motivation and good intentions will result in failure if not preceded by careful and purposeful planning. This section will provide you with guidance regarding factors concerning your exercise road trip.

Weighing In

It is not unusual to weigh in on a daily basis. The scales should be on a non-carpeted surface, and you must be consistent in what you are wearing.

The weigh-in should be in the morning before eating and exercising. Keep a record of the daily weights as well as having a section for comments regarding the previous day's events. These may include unusual eating behaviors, specific exercise types (weights, treadmill, etc.), water intake, illness, and so forth.

You may be surprised to see all of what can affect your weight. It won't take long to see patterns develop that may prompt you to alter your exercise program or to change your dietary habits.

There are many factors that can affect weight changes; and the older we get, it seems like most of these may be the result of weight gains. Some include a reduction in general activity, medication side effects, water retention, diet, and in a lowering of your metabolic rate.

However, if your daily routine hasn't changed, but suddenly you begin to lose weight, consider this to be a warning sign, and get it checked out.

Scales have come a long way over the past decades, and I suspect that many of you may still be clinging to the needle type. By now, the adjustment screw is nearly worn out. It's time for you to join the digital-scale age. These have read-outs in big, bold letters with less than pound increments. Some also have a body-fat-index component, although I question their accuracy.

A gradual onset of balance issues may result in weight gains. Being fearful of losing our balance, there is a tendency not to be as active and to eat more. As the abdominal cavity becomes larger, the more anterior is the center of gravity, meaning we could have a tendency to lose our balances in the forward direction. Therefore, one of the goals of an exercise program may be to lose weight.

Don't exercise so you can eat more. It is easy to outeat any workout with regards to calories. Keep in mind that exercises to improve balance may take time and that weight loss may be a byproduct, not the ultimate goal.

THE IMPORTANCE OF WATER

Why not more water? Why don't we Seniors drink at least eight 8 oz. glasses of water every day? Consider the following excuses:

1. Water doesn't taste good.
2. I prefer sodas.
3. My eight cups of coffee each day should count for water intake as well.
4. I retain water, so I drink as little as I can.
5. My joints hurt too much to stand and walk to the kitchen.
6. I'm too tired to get a drink.
7. I'm not thirsty; I'm hungry.
8. I can't remember to drink more.
9. The more water that goes in, the more that comes out.

Why more water? What you don't know may hurt you. Compare the following list with the previous one. Drinking more water is not only a good idea; it is a necessity, especially for the Senior crowd.

1. The average adult body contains 55%-75% water, and 75% of Americans are chronically dehydrated.
2. Even mild dehydration will slow down your metabolism as much as 3%.
3. In 37% of Americans, the body's thirst mechanism is so weak that it is often mistaken for hunger.
4. In a University of Washington study, 98% of dieters' hunger pangs were deterred by one glass of water.
5. The biggest trigger of daytime fatigue is the lack of water.
6. Spinal discs and joint cartilage have high water content. The body will draw water from these areas when dehydrated causing many spine and joint ailments.
7. Preliminary research findings indicate that eight to ten glasses of water a day could ease back and joint pain for up to 80% of sufferers.
8. All the bodily systems rely on water to function properly, including digestion, food absorption, regulation of body temperature, transportation of nutrients and oxygen to cells, and for the removal of toxins and other wastes.
9. When a body fails to take in sufficient water to function properly, it will retain what water it has.
10. Conversely, the more water that is consumed, the less is retained.
11. Caffeine is a diuretic; the more that is consumed, even greater is the water that is excreted through urine. Caffeine also depletes vitamin C.
12. Urinary incontinence is a common problem that can be helped by certain exercises. Withholding water will only make it worse.

Consider some of the contributing factors for balance problems, fatigue, sore joints, muscle pain, and mental dullness. Then imagine what positive effects eight glasses of water a day could have on the overall state of your health. Water, an inexpensive wonder "drug" with no negative side effects, imagine that!

You can fit drinking those eight glasses into your other rituals—at meals, when you brush your teeth, or when you take vitamins or medications and when you exercise.

SHOULD I MONITOR MY BLOOD PRESSURE AND HEART RATE?

This is between you and your physician; however, keep in mind that there are many factors influencing blood pressure, and exercise is only one. Compare the blood pressure reading from your physician visit with those at your local pharmacy's do-it-yourself machines. They should be close.

Now eliminate all caffeine and drink eight glasses of water a day for two weeks then recheck it. That will probably do more good for your blood pressure than stretching and strengthening.

Aerobic exercises like the treadmill and bike riding, etc., may provide some positive blood pressure results in the long run. Also, if you no longer are worried about losing your balance, this means less stress.

HOW HARD SHOULD I WORK OUT?

The gold standard for measuring the optimal tolerance to exercise is the target heart rate. By monitoring our heart rates, we are able to determine our body's responses to exercise and to limit the intensity of the workouts before our hearts are overly stressed.

Seniors are urged to reach their own target rate gradually, particularly if they have been pretty much sedentary. Most Seniors should aim no higher than 70 to 85 percent of the maximum rate listed.

The recommended ranges for heart rates (beats per minute) for Seniors are:

Age	Heart Rate (bpm)
60	112-136
70	105-128

80	98-119
90	91-111
100	84-102

Taking Your Pulse. This isn't difficult, but it can be tricky. The tip of the index and middle fingers is placed against the inside of the opposite wrist, just below the mound at the base of the thumb. Count the throbs for twenty seconds and multiply by three to get the heart rate for one minute. If you have been relatively inactive for five minutes this is your resting heart rate.

The radial pulse is sometimes difficult to locate, but try each wrist before giving up. An alternative location is beside the Adam's apple. Press gently with the index and middle finger tips, but don't push so hard that you compromise the blood flow and get light headed.

Another option is to purchase a heart rate monitor for about $250 or buy one as an option on a treadmill.

Aerobic exercises. Brisk walking or running, treadmill, and biking condition the heart and lungs by increasing the efficiency of oxygen intake by the body. Although aerobic exercise is probably a good idea, many Seniors with balance issues will improve without doing them.

For those who choose to do an aerobic activity, monitoring your heart rate is mandatory. This is so you don't exceed your target heart rate, and it provides you with an objective method of assessing recovery time.

Midway into your moderate aerobic exercise, take your pulse. If you are in the midrange or lower on your heart rate scale, finish the activity then retake your pulse. The heart rate should increase but it should take no more than three to five minutes to get the pulse back down to the resting heart rate. If it takes longer than that to recover, you overdid it.

Regardless of what new exercise or activity you decide to do, you may feel okay right afterward, but a couple hours later you experience weakness or a sick sensation. Chances are, you may have over stressed your system and should cut back the intensity for a while. If the pain, weakness, or ill sensations don't go away, check with a physician.

The Importance of Proper Breathing

Long hours of an inactive lifestyle combined with rounded shoulder posture promotes shallow breathing, decreased blood oxygenation, and generalized fatigue. This goes for couch potatoes of all ages, the computer addicts as well as for the sedentary Seniors.

The primary muscle of respiration is the diaphragm, and, like all muscles, it will weaken if not challenged.

To recondition the diaphragm, lie on your back on a firm surface with your knees bent and a small pillow under your head. Breathe in for five counts and slowly exhale for ten seconds resisting the flow with semitight (pursed) lips.

Do five to ten times or fewer if you get light headed. Do three sets several times a day. For a greater challenge, place a heavy book or weight on your abdomen, and lift it upward as you breathe in.

The importance of breathing while lifting weights is well documented. However, it is equally necessary to incorporate a regular breathing pattern into your aerobic activities.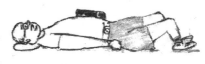

When dancing, I often concentrate on posture and technique so intensely that I hold my breath. When this happens, the body is using oxygen but failing to replenish it.

The consequences of improper breathing were brought to national awareness in the 2007 *Dancing With The Stars* competition. Marie Osmond had just completed a dance. As she was awaiting the judges' comments, she fainted because she forgot to breathe.

Seniors may also have a contributing factor not commonly associated with the younger crowd, and that is hardening of the arteries and impaired circulation. Failure to sufficiently oxygenate the blood through efficient breathing could result in issues affecting balance and stability.

What is the Proper Dress for Exercising?

If wearing your school colors or a matching outfit motivates you to exercise, go for it. Otherwise, the one major guideline is to wear clothing that does not restrict movement. Also, do not use those rubber or vinyl suits once promoted to encourage you to sweat. The skin needs to breathe and to perspire.

Shoes or no shoes are individual choices. For some activities, being barefoot promotes the strengthening of the individual foot muscles and joints. A walking program, on the other hand, requires shoes fitted to the person and designed for walking. Never buy those shoes at a garage sale. Once a person has worn a pair of shoes, the sole becomes molded for that person.

Shoe wear may be a matter of necessity, comfort, or stability. Do what is best for you and your situation.

WHAT WAS THAT CHAPTER ALL ABOUT?

How often have we heard the statement that it is the little things that count? That is what this chapter is all about. You may be so anxious to improve your balance that you are perhaps willing to ignore some really good suggestions just to get started sooner.

There is no justification so great as to override commonsense. Your weight, drinking plenty of water, whether to monitor your blood pressure, how hard you work out, proper breathing, and wearing exercise clothing that doesn't restrict movements are all important.

Chapter 21

Exercise Guidelines

Individual needs and resources will dictate which approach is initially taken or ultimately pursued. This section deals with the finer points of an exercise program. Keep in mind that guidelines are always subject to modification. If in doubt as to how aggressive you should be, always start with the least intense level and then gradually progress only as you feel comfortable in doing so.

How Important is Speed in Exercising?

If you need to visualize the ideal speed of an exercise, consider Tai Chi. Imagine a Chinese park early in the morning. Young and old perform a series of choreographed movements with grace and control. There is no reward for those who finish first, and no one is in respiratory distress. You observe a calm environment and a general sense of accomplishment.

When it comes to exercise, one of the most difficult principles to get across is that slower is better. The reasons apply to all ages but especially for Seniors who seem to take longer to recover from injuries.

Slow lifts and stretches are more effective and safer, plus they require a greater amount of control. Observe how balance-impaired Seniors walk. They take short strikes and fast steps because they are unable to maintain balance at slower paces.

This "slow" philosophy will pay big dividends.

WHY IS EXACT FORM SO IMPORTANT?

As you gain proficiency in style, performance levels will show gains based more on proper form than on changes in your physiology. For this reason, keep in mind that practice does not make perfect. Only perfect practice makes perfect. Imperfect practice makes imperfect. My daughter's gymnastic coach reminded her of this on a regular basis.

Proper form is the best way to assure that what you are targeting in your exercise is exactly what is being challenged. Efficiency in function translates into fewer extraneous movements, enhanced control, less fatigue, and, ultimately, in better balance. It's not just about form; it's *all* about form.

WHEN SHOULD I EXERCISE?

If there was an ideal time, the health clubs would be overwhelmed for a couple hours and empty the rest of the day.

Employment responsibilities dictated when you could work out, but now in retirement you have choices. It's okay to be flexible in the scheduling of your exercise program as long as you adhere to "The Rules."

Rule #1: Any exercise pursued before breakfast should be restricted to those done while lying down or sitting. Your blood sugar should be relatively low because of the eight hours or so of fasting. Eat a light breakfast and wait about a half hour before getting into aerobics or strengthening. Stretching can begin while still in bed and balancing right after breakfast.

Rule # 2: Never exercise after over eating. Better yet, never over eat. Focus on why you are eating, and it is not for hibernation. When exercising, your body needs to be hydrated (water) and requires fuel (food) and not coffee and sweet rolls. Smaller meals and eating more frequently merits consideration.

Rule #3: Exercise during the same time period each day (mid-morning, mid-afternoon, or early evening). Once a routine is established, the body will adapt to it and anticipate it. This goes for sleep, eating, and exercising.

How Many Repetitions (Reps) Should I Do?

Reps are the number of times you do one particular activity in succession. Reps usually refer to stretches or lifts. Since both exercises will be performed slowly and with good form, a five-to-ten repetition maximum is advised.

Even when an activity is new to you, if you can't do five reps, your resistance is too great.

How Many Sets?

A set is the five to ten reps you just completed. Three sets are sufficient for strengthening exercises and stretches.

How Long Should Rests Between Sets Be?

When doing resistance exercises, there must be a rest period between sets to permit the muscles to recover before the next set. Thirty seconds is the recommended standard. However, you can be creative with this rest period. If you are doing right leg lifts, complete one set, and, during the rest, do left leg lifts. Stretches can also be a productive "rest." For Seniors, a sixty-second purposeful rest period will not distract from the effectiveness of the exercise.

If, on the other hand, you want a super-charged strengthening program, here is what Joe Dowdell, president of Peak Performance Strength & Conditioning Center in New York suggests. Spend less time between sets at the beginning of the workout when the muscles aren't tired and more time toward the end of the workout. He calls this density training. He says it makes the muscles work harder and at the same time improves endurance. I'm tired just thinking about it.

How Long Should I Hold?

In the middle of every exercise you find the word AHOLD."

You shouldn't let those HOLDs slide by unnoticed. They are an important part of the exercise. The length of these HOLDs will vary depending on the exercise you are doing.

Isotonic strengthening occurs when there is joint movement around which the muscles are working. At the peak of the "lift," do an Olympic hold. That is a brief period that demonstrates that you have control.

For isometric strengthening (no movement), *hold* fifteen seconds. When actively stretching, use a thirty-second *hold*. A passive stretch, such as leaning forward to stretch the calves, should be done slowly and carefully with a sixty-second *hold*. After a week or so of faithfully doing your *holds*, you will know how long to *hold* without counting.

Isolating the muscle or muscle group will enhance the effectiveness of the exercise. Feel the tension of the stretch. During the lift and *hold*, think about the muscle being targeted rather than just going through the motions mechanically.

How Heavy Should the Weights Be?

Chances are that any weight will be more challenging than what you are using now. As you complete your reps and sets, you will experience that "momentary muscle fatigue"; after which time, proper form is compromised if you continue without rest.

If you felt no fatigue, you can add more resistance. If you couldn't complete ten reps, you used too much weight.

Rating the intensity of an exercise or activity is subjective because of the varying fitness levels of each participant. For this reason, we have the Borg scale to refer to.

The Borg Scale

Exertion Level	Functional Level
6 Least effort	At Rest
7 Very, Very Light	
8 9 Very Light 10	
11 Fairly Light 12 13 Somewhat Hard 14	Levels 11-14 are the Endurance Training Zone
15 Hard 16 17 Very Hard 18 19	Levels 15-17 are the Strength Training Zone
20	Running for a Bus

So it sounds like what the experts are saying is, "You Seniors, go figure it out for yourselves," which makes some sense. Seniors beginning an exercise program will probably want to aim at what is, to them, "very light" and work up to what seems "somewhat hard."

The best advice is to start low and to increase to tolerance. Add no more than ten percent per week—that's true of weights or repetitions. Also, if you cannot equal or exceed the weight levels and reps from your last workout, you have not yet recovered.

How Long Before I See Results?

You will see remarkable strength gains in a couple weeks if for no reason than becoming familiar with the exercises. On the other hand, one session of overly aggressive stretching or too-vigorous strengthening, may set you back two weeks.

Arm muscles generally get stronger faster, and the ankle, calf, and the toes are the hardest to get back in shape. Could this be attributed to the higher degree of circulation and oxygenation in the arm versus the legs?

What Was That Chapter All About?

Seniors with balance issues often also have strength deficits. Failure to address this will prolong recovery. Variables to consider are when you should exercise, how many reps and sets, the rests and *holds*, how heavy the weights should be, how hard you should exercise, and how soon you will see results.

Chapter 22

THE IMPORTANCE OF POSTURE

Before we begin discussing stretching, strengthening, and balancing exercises, we need to recognize the importance of posture in all our daily activities and in our exercise program.

Bad posture is, I believe, at the heart of many of our balance problems.

Posture is important to all Seniors but especially for those who are unsteady. We get in the habit of leaning forward and when we do, it throws our center of gravity forward, causing imbalance. Think about that the next time you stare at the ground as you walk.

In my professional life, I have admired perfect posture, and, conversely, I have come to the realization that many ill-defined syndromes, like progressive unsteadiness, have been preceded by a lifestyle of compromised postures.

In this chapter, posture will be defined; you will be given the opportunity for self assessment, and you will be further enlightened as to the importance of posture.

WHAT IS POSTURE?

Posture is the attitude of the body; a fairly simple statement for a very complex concept. When the term "posture" is brought up, many Seniors will reflect back to their elementary years when good posture was assessed by the ability to stand and to walk around with a book on the top of the head. I recently returned from the Caribbean and took a picture of a lady carrying a large fruit basket on her head. We don't see that around here!

Posture principles are not only when walking or sitting, but also when reclining. Do you read or watch TV in bed with your head propped forward? This is poor posture.

Do you drive with you seat too far forward or too far back? Do you sleep on your back with your head held excessively elevated? These are not acceptable postures.

HOW TO ASSESS CORRECT POSTURE

The American Physical Therapy Association recommends the following self test. Stand with your back against a wall, feet shoulder width apart and three to six inches from the wall. Your arms should be at the sides. Press the head, shoulders, and back against the wall. Now, push the belly button back toward the spine taking the arch out of the back. Next, push away from the wall with your elbows keeping the back straight. If you are able to do all this, you have good posture.

Another way to check your postural alignment is to stand upright looking straight ahead. A vertical line should intersect the cheek bones, the breast bone or sternum, and the pubic bone. If so, back up against a wall and the back of the head, the shoulders, and the buttocks should touch at the same time.

Now that you have assessed your upright posture, can you sustain it? If so, with a concentrated effort and input from those around you, (Straighten up!) your new and improved posture will feel more normal in a couple months.

If you are only able to make a partial correction, do it! This may prevent an otherwise-progressive deformity. If you want to have fun while improving your posture, try ballroom dancing.

BREATHING AND POSTURE

The diaphragm is located below the lungs and acts as a transverse divider between the chest and the abdominal cavity. As a breath is taken in, the diaphragm lowers creating negative pressure in the chest cavity. Air rushes into the lungs through the nose and/or mouth to equalize the pressure. As the diaphragm drops, the abdomen expands to make room.

Chest breathing. Some of you may challenge this saying that the abdomen draws in as you breathe in, and it is your chest that expands. This is chest breathing which is incorrect, inefficient, and fatiguing.

Watch a baby breathe while asleep on his/her back, or gently put your hand on the baby's abdomen. The tummy rises with each breath (inhalation).

When sitting or bending at the waist, the abdominal contents are compressed and restricted in their ability to expand. This promotes shallow breathing resulting in compromised blood oxygenation. This can lead to fatigue, dizziness, and mental dullness.

The trained vocalist will stand with good posture to enhance breath control. Do you have shortness of breath? Learn to breathe more efficiently.

Excessive Sitting

Medical conditions leading to balance issues can begin with excessive sitting. We have been made aware that being restricted to a seat while flying compromises circulation to the legs. Yet people spend hours at a time mesmerized by video screens.

On planes, we complain because we can't easily get up and walk around, but, at home or work, we get so engrossed that we don't get up. The result is the same: impaired lower extremity circulation. While temporary at first, over the years, the condition becomes permanent.

Did you ever sit so long and still that your leg or foot went to sleep? Pressure on the sciatic nerve in your buttocks can do that. People at times try to walk it off only to lose their balance and at times fall.

Bad posture and losing your balance. Looking upward or even straight ahead while in a forward head posture (sitting or standing), can pinch the structures at the base of your skull. The early symptoms can be headaches, or you can go directly to getting dizzy or passing out.

The ramifications of a forward leaning posture is that the body's center of gravity is anterior, that is further forward than where it should be, which could result in two responses. One is that the back muscles will work harder to keep you upright. These muscles can become painful and eventually fatigued to the degree that they fail to hold you up and you lean forward even more.

The second is a tendency to fall forward. Compensation is to walk faster to keep ahead of the fall. Catch a toe, and you are down.

Canes will support the postural muscles and help keep you from falling forward. Walkers, on the other hand, encourage you to lean forward just to hold the handles.

When doing balance tests later on and you consistently lean to the front, your problem could be a forward-leaning posture. Have someone observe you from the side to get his/her input.

POSTURAL MANAGEMENT TECHNIQUES

You know how to assess your posture, and for some, the transformation from bad to better posture may just be awareness and practice. Those with the best prognosis are the ones who are getting progressively worse but can still straighten up when they think about it.

For others, correction will include stretching tight structures, strengthening overstretched, weak muscles, and incorporating breathing into certain exercises.

In the advanced stages of conditions like Ankylosing Spondylitis and scoliosis, the spine becomes fused. The exercises I can recommend will be helpful only while the spine still retains some mobility. They will not help those with fused spines.

NORMAL SPINAL CURVATURE

The normal spinal curvatures are an arched neck, a slightly rounded upper back, and a mildly swayed low back. Medically speaking, these are cervical lordosis, thoracic kyphosis, and lumbar lordosis. Put all together, the spine makes an *S* curve.

Sitting in a slouched position changes the *S* curve into a *C* curve. The neck becomes forward, the upper back rounds even more, and the lower back flattens out. Sitting, such as when you are at the computer, riding in a car, watching TV, reading, etc., encourages this *C* curve posture.

Another *C* curve occurs when we curl up on our sides when sleeping. In time, it becomes progressively more difficult to stand straight, and we develop the forward lean posture. The greater the "lean," is the more likely the chances for balance problems.

WHAT WAS THAT CHAPTER ALL ABOUT?

Posture is defined and tests are given to determine your posture. Breathing and posture, the effects of excessive sitting, and bad posture are described. Postural management techniques and normal spinal curvature are addressed.

Chapter 23

RESTORATIVE POSTURAL TECHNIQUES

Garfield reportedly once said, "What I like to do best is nothing, and then take a nap afterward." Correcting your posture while doing "nothing" is a great concept, and it works.

PRONE LYING

Take one or more time-outs during the day to lie flat on your stomach. You can also assume this position when you go to bed and before you get up. How long in this position depends on how it feels, but fifteen minutes at a time should work well. For me, this is not a particularly comfortable way to lie, but it does feel good when I get up.

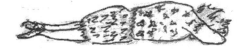

LUMBAR SUPPORTS

Couches, chairs, and car seats were not all created equally. What is an ideal fit for one family member is a total misfit for another.

A seat too deep encourages a person to scoot out so that the knees can bend at the edge. The result is no low back support and a C curved spine. A small pillow behind the back will support the lumbar curve, and you sit up straighter.

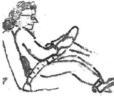 Car seats have the same potential for sustaining poor posture. If the seat needs to be closer to the wheel, adjust it and then engage the built in lumbar support, roll up a towel, use a small pillow, or buy a custom-made lumbar device.

Once you find the perfect support, the hours you spend in a car seat become therapeutic.

READING POSTURE

If you choose to read in bed, do it correctly. Support the entire back with a wedge of pillows rather than lying relatively flat and pushing your head forward.

In addition to the lumbar support in your reading chair, use a foot stool and prop your arms on a pillow. This elevates your reading material rather than bending your neck to your book.

DYNAMIC POSTURAL STRETCHES

We can target three regions of the body in which we can correct posture—the cervical, the lumbar, and the chest areas.

Reducing the head-jutting posture can prevent dizziness and counteract the tendency to lean forward. Restoring lumbar lordosis will assist in standing more upright. Improving chest mobility will permit enhanced respiration and upper body posture.

Cervical glides. The cervical spine (neck) is the most vulnerable of all the spinal segments. It's not surrounded by internal organs or other bony structures but just "sits" on the shoulders like a twelve-pound ball. As the head and neck jut forward, the twelve-pound head creates 24-48-pound forces on the neck joints. Maintaining this position long enough can result in pinched nerves, disc problems, headaches, and fatigued muscles.

The space between the base of the skull and the first cervical vertebra gets pinched as do the structures that pass through this area. The result can be dizziness and possibly fainting.

Cervical glides attempt to reposition the head from the forward position to one more on top of the body.

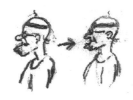

Put two fingers on the front of the chin just below the lip. Gently guide the head back without tilting the head. The eyes always will be looking straight ahead. Maintain this posture when standing, walking, and sitting. If you must look down, do the cervical glide and then look down with your chin, not the neck.

Lumbar extension. Taking frequent breaks from sitting is a good idea. This includes in the home, office, motor vehicle, etc. Stand with your feet shoulder width apart and slowly straighten up. Place your hands on the pelvic bones and gently push forward increasing the low back curve.

Hold fifteen to thirty seconds (longer if you like), and do as many as you feel comfortable with. You may feel resistance, but you don't want to continue if you experience pain.

Incorporate this stretch into your daily routine especially after sitting. Do not sit longer than one half hour without stretching. Break up extended road trips with frequent stretch breaks. Stretch before you climb into bed. Be gentle as you "unwind," and don't forget to breathe when stretching. Don't hold your breath.

Chest expansion. If you fail the tight pectorals test (testing in the flexibility chapter 24), this exercise is especially for you. Stand with your upper arms and forearms horizontal to the floor with your finger tips touching. Slowly bring your

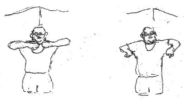

elbows out to the sides. As you do this, take in a five-second chest breath.

At the end range or the *hold*, pinch your shoulder blades together. Slowly breathe out as you return to the starting position. The goal is to do five in a row providing you don't get dizzy from hyperventilating. The reason for the chest breath, instead of the abdominal breath, is to use the air entering the chest cavity to assist with chest expansion from the inside.

Corner stretches can be effective chest mobilizers. Stand facing a corner with your upper arms horizontal to the floor, elbows slightly extended, and finger tips pointing upward. Slowly lean into the corner, *hold* and return. If this seems too easy or you don't feel a pulling sensation across the chest, gradually adjust the hand position so that the fingers eventually point directly into the corner.

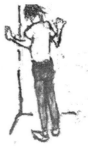

UPPER BACK STRENGTHENING

Years of rounded shoulder posture lead to overstretched and weakened rhomboid muscles. These muscles are located in the midback region and function to retract the shoulder blades.

Stretching the tight chest region will do little good if the rhomboids aren't strong enough to sustain an upright posture. The following are options for strengthening the rhomboids.

Rowing machines will target the rhomboids, but I don't like the position you must assume. Instead, see if the fitness center has a machine where you sit with your back unsupported and pull on two hand grips.

If so, go easy on the resistance. Row slowly and concentrate on form and technique. Sit tall (straight back), pull slowly, and when you get to the *hold*, pinch the shoulder blades together. Does this sound familiar?

Home rowing can be accomplished using elastic bands or tubes. Tie a knot in the middle and shut a door on it so you're on one side and the knot is on the other side. If you have a support pole in your basement, use it for an anchor.

You may sit or stand, but the shoulder blades must be free to move, and the resistance is coming from the band anchored directly in front of the chest. Tie loops for handles. Use the same form and technique as you would on a rowing machine. Resistance can be varied by how much tension is applied to the band.

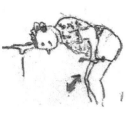

Dumbbell rows strengthen one rhomboid at a time. The technique involves bending forward, supporting, yourself on the left arm or forearm so that the right arm is free to dangle. Raise the right elbow up and out to the side as far as it will go. The forearm and hand remain pointing to the floor. Then pinch the right shoulder blade toward the spine on the *hold*. Return slowly to the dangle to complete one rep.

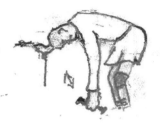

Begin with no resistance until you are comfortable with the form and technique. Add resistance using dumbbells or anything else of relatively light weight. Do five reps with the right arm before doing five with the left. Remember to breathe when rowing, and be aware that you may experience some dizziness upon standing.

SOME SIMPLE THINGS YOU CAN DO TO IMPROVE YOUR POSTURE

1. Walk tall with your shoulders held slightly back.
2. When seated, place a pillow or a rolled towel in the small of your back.
3. When lying down, use a pillow to support your head and neck but not to force yourself into awkward positions.

WHAT WAS THAT CHAPTER ALL ABOUT?

There is much to consider regarding posture and postural stresses. I equate abnormal posture as being the hub of a wheel where the tire is a composite of symptoms. Postural awareness is the first step in rehab. The second involves specific postural exercises. The third is that every minute that you stretch, lift a weight, walk, etc., you are not in a static sitting posture.

Working on correcting poor posture is work. It takes time, dedication, and effort. Incorporating postural principles into all phases of your activities of daily or nightly living will become the keystone of your balance program.

Later when you do balance tests, observe the postures you assume when doing them. Now, get comfortable with your new and improved posture, retake the tests, and be prepared to be pleasantly surprised at the results.

Chapter 24

TESTING YOUR FLEXIBILITY

IS ALL STRETCHING HELPFUL?

To stretch or not to stretch; that is the question. As a physical therapist for over forty years, I have seen both the benefits of carefully planned flexibility programs as well as the disasters from well-intentioned but overly aggressive stretches.

As a reminder, we Seniors are not as flexible as our junior counterparts. Progressive inactivity along with decades of poor nutritional input, combined with the natural aging process, specifically degenerating joints and spines, have promoted a sedentary lifestyle. As our bodies age, the progressive tightness occurring in some areas may actually be the body's natural way of protecting itself from injury.

So we don't need to stretch? Not so! The beneficial effects of stretching are for all ages. These include the prevention and reduction of musculoskeletal pain, the improvement of posture, the enhancement of the respiratory system, and the lessening of the risk of tripping and losing your balance.

FLEXIBILITY ASSESSMENT KEY AREAS

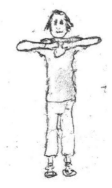

Pectoral muscles. Rounded shoulders and forward head posture are common companions with tight chest muscles. This forward lean can result in an anterior center of gravity, putting you at risk for losing your balance forward. Chest tightness can also lead to progressive breathing difficulties.

To test for tight chest muscles, stand with your upper arms and forearms horizontal to the floor and with your finger tips touching. Slowly bring your elbows out to the sides. If you are unable to extend them past your midline, you are tight.

Hip Flexors. Hip flexor tightness can contribute to a tendency to lose your balance in the forward direction and to walk with short, shuffle steps.

Lie flat on your back with both legs straight. Bring one knee up, and pull the bent leg from the thigh toward your chest using both arms. If you cannot maintain surface contact with the bottom leg, you have tight hip flexors on that side. Then repeat with the opposite leg. The secondary effect of tight hip flexors can be a forward leaning posture, back pain, and a tendency to lose your balance.

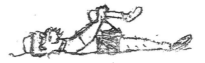

Calf muscles. Heel cords are the tendons that attach the calf muscles to the calcaneus (heel) bones. We speak of tight heel cords, but, in reality, it is the inflexibility in the calf muscles that can cause you to catch your toe as you attempt to take a step. Before you know it, you are shuffling your feet. As the tightness gets worse, the greater chance there is of tripping, losing your balance forward, and falling.

To check for tightness, stand facing a wall. Touch the wall with both hands. Bend the left knee, which is directly under you, and place your right toes back about eight to twelve inches. Gradually push the heel toward the floor. If you can't, you have a tight heel cord. Repeat the test with the opposite foot.

WHAT WAS THAT CHAPTER ALL ABOUT?

Physical therapists and other health-care professionals may prescribe stretching exercises to counteract specific syndromes. There are even entire books on stretching for practically every muscle in the body. However, I chose three muscle groups that often become tight in Seniors. Tightness in them can compromise balance and increase the risk of falling.

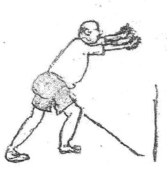

Chapter 25

GUIDELINES FOR
STRETCHING EXERCISES

The purpose of this chapter is to explore the subject of stretching for balance-challenged Seniors, not to critique stretching techniques for other Senior disorders. However, the principles to follow apply to all stretches.

TIGHTNESS IN SENIORS

Inflexibility in Seniors is often the main source of stability. Muscular tightness is the result of the body adapting to decades of insidious changes brought about by inactivity or abuse. For example, tight hamstrings may have resulted from years of excessive sitting for one individual while, in another, the hamstring tightness may have slowly developed to provide stability in a knee injured years before. Indiscriminate stretching, however well-intended, could have negative ramifications.

RANGE OF MOTION (ROM)

Range of motion is the degree of mobility available by a structure articulating about a joint. For example, an arm hanging down at the side is at 0E of shoulder flexion. However, when that same extremity is raised to the front and directly overhead, the ROM is 180 degrees of flexion. Each joint has these assigned numbers or degrees indicating its normal ROM.

Loss of ROM. ROM is compromised by inactivity (includes sleeping), injury, arthritis, and water retention to name a few. If you have an opportunity, watch a cat that is taking a nap all curled up in a ball. Upon awakening, it goes into a full-body extension stretch.

This is a natural process instinctively performed to provide relief and prepare for activity. For that matter, babies stretch when they wake up. I wonder when we stopped doing that!

The loss of ROM can be reflected in altered body mechanics, how we walk, postural adaptations, and in impaired balance.

The section on "Stretching in Bed" is intended as a wake-up program for your muscles and joints. Guidelines for these stretches differ somewhat from those directed at mobilizing tight structures, although some principles apply to both. These stretches, in many cases, also double as ROM exercises.

Guidelines for stretching include:

1. Proceed slowly with each motion.
2. Hold for a five (5) count.
3. Do three reps.
4. Hold longer and do more reps on the structures that are tighter and that are responding positively to your efforts.
5. Never stretch to create pain or through pain.
6. Assume that if you are instructed to do an exercise with one arm, leg, foot, etc., that you are "next to do it with the other."

There may be an instance where a particular stretch, properly applied, yields undesirable results. Will you know when to stop? You may stretch a structure that doesn't need stretching. Will you be able to recognize this? There may be more than one technique available to stretch the same structure. Will you be able to determine what works for you? You may be too aggressive when stretching. Will you be able to ease up?

How Much Tension Should I Feel During a Stretch?

For years, my response was to go as far as you can then a little bit farther. Perhaps a more humane response is to feel a gentle tension, going up to the point of discomfort, and then holding. Use minimal force or strain, and *no* bouncing.

It is not unusual for the muscle being stretched to become tense. If you feel this happening, let up on the stretch and resume after it has relaxed. If it doesn't, you may be overstretching. You want to be able to say, "I feel the stretch, but it doesn't hurt."

What Was That Chapter All About?

Inflexibility in Seniors is often their main source of stability. This chapter gives guidelines for increasing range of motion and how much tenseness should be felt in a stretch.

Chapter 26

STRETCHING EXERCISES

STRETCHING IN BED

Hands, wrists, and elbows. Bend both elbows and wrists, make fists, and turn palms toward you. Extend both elbows and wrists as you open the hands, spread the fingers, and turn palms away.

Arm raises. Lie on your back, clasp both hands, and raise your arms to where they are pointing toward the ceiling. Slowly go up and down, side-to-side and in circles one way then the other.

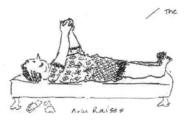

VARIATIONS:

1. One arm at a time or together but without clasping.
2. Clasp the hands and continue to go over your head, bending the elbows and ending up with the hands at the top of the head.

Ankle Alphabet. Lie on your back, resting the right calf on top of the left shin so the right ankle is free to move. Spell out the alphabet with your big toe while moving the right ankle but not the leg. You may do it more than once if you like.

VARIATIONS:

1. Print or write the alphabet in either uppercase or lowercase letters.

2. Write out the count to twenty-six.

Heel cords. These are the tendons that attach the calf muscles to the calcaneus (heel) bones. Tightness can prevent you from fully clearing your toes underneath you as you step. Before you know it, you are shuffling your feet. The tighter the heel cords, the greater is the risk of falling and losing your balance forward.

Lie on your back with knees straight and bend toes toward your knees (ankle dorsiflexion). Tense the quads (muscles on top of thigh). Slowly return and gently point your toes. *Caution:* Do not be too aggressive with the toe pointing as this may cause calf cramps.

Heel slides. Lie on your back with both legs straight. Slide the right heel toward the buttocks while remaining in contact with the bed. *Hold* at the high point and slowly return.

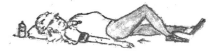

Hamstring stretches. Hamstring tightness has been blamed as a contributing factor for a number of musculoskeletal syndromes. On the other hand, in my physical therapy practice, numerous clients were identified as having tight hamstrings, but this was of no clinical significance regarding their complaints.

However, my mission is to inform and to educate you and not to encourage or discourage you from doing hamstring stretches.

Demonstrating Option 3:

If you choose to include hamstring stretches, or any stretch, into your ROM or rehabilitation program, you may need to experiment with a variety of positions and techniques that give you the desired results without creating new problems.

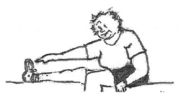

In this section, the hamstring stretches are to be done on a bed, but could be adapted for other locations.

Option 1: Lie on your back with both knees bent and feet flat. Bring the right knee toward you so you are able to clasp your hands behind the thigh just below the knee. Extend the right leg, *hold,* and return. If you do not feel any "pulling" behind your right thigh, repeat but this time bring the right knee closer to your chest and straighten your leg so that the foot is pointing more overhead. As a bonus, this is also a gentle abdominal strengthening exercise.

Option 2: Sit on the edge of the bed with both legs dangling. It's okay if the feet touch the floor. Lean back and support your body with both arms. Slowly extend the right leg completely and *hold.* If the "pulling" sensation is too great behind the thigh to fully extend, try to lean back farther. However, if you feel little or no "pulling," sit more erect or forward.

Option 3: Sit on the edge of a bed with your right leg on the bed fully extended. The left leg is bent with the foot touching the floor. Hold on to the right leg with both hands and slowly pull your chest toward the right knee and hold.

Hip abduction. Lie on your back with your legs together and straight. Spread them apart as far as you can and at the same time. Make sure that the knee caps and toes do not roll outward when spreading, and maintain a straight back the entire time.

Hip rotation. Lie on your back with your legs straight but slightly apart and with your toes pointed up. Roll your feet and knees outward so the toes are pointing more to the side. Keep the legs straight and roll them inward so the toes of each foot are pointing toward each other. *Hold* at the extremes of each roll.

Variation: Lie on your back, knees bent, and feet apart. Roll the knees out and entire time then in. Keep your feet touching the bed the entire time!

Back stretches. Lie on your back with knees bent. Grab hold of the right thigh under the knee with both hands and pull it toward your chest. *Hold* and slowly return, but don't let go. Repeat several times, especially if you are relaxing with more with each pull. This is also referred to as "Knee to Chest."

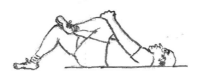

Variation: Lie on your back with knees bent and legs together. Clasp your thighs and draw them toward your chest. *Hold* and slowly return but don't let go. Repeat several times if you are gaining mobility. Stop immediately if this causes or aggravates sciatic-type symptoms. This exercise is also referred to as "Double Knee to Chest."

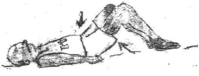

Variation: Lie on your back with knees bent and arms at your sides. Press the small of your back into the bed, tightening the muscles of your abdomen and buttocks. Once you feel comfortable with this method, repeat with your legs straight. *Hold* at the point where you feel the back flattening. This exercise is also known as the "Pelvic Tilt."

Variation: Kneel on hands and knees distributing your weight evenly. Lower your head as you raise your back. Then raise your head and sway your back. Avoid if you have knee, wrist, hand, or other problems getting into the starting position.

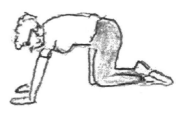

Back-and-Hip Stretch. Lie on your back with both knees bent and feet touching the bed. Cross your right thigh over your left thigh. Turn your head to the right, and extend your right arm straight out to the right. Slip your left hand between your thighs clasping the right thigh. Gently pull the right knee toward the left shoulder. *Hold* and slowly return. *Do not do this exercise if you have had total hip or hip prosthesis surgery.*

Bridging or Body Raise. Lie on your back, knees bent, feet flat, and arms straight either at your sides or slightly away from your body. Lift your buttocks off the surface of the bed. You can *hold* thirty seconds or, if you can't, try something like this: work up to thirty repetitions, with one-to-two-second *holds*, raising your buttocks a little bit at first and progressively higher. Do not strain, and do not hold your breath when bridging.

ADDITIONAL STRETCHES

A specific stretch targets a defined muscle or muscle group, but rarely are the tight structures elongated without compromising others. Muscles do not stand alone. They are linked by 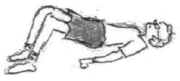 numerous connective tissues and joints, some of which have greater extensibility. A stretch applied to one muscle or muscle group will transfer its effect to the loosest link in the chain. The result can be that what was tight remains tight and what was loose gets looser.

When at all possible, attempt to stabilize adjacent structures when stretching others. Some stretches have been omitted because of this.

In this section, we will assume that certain structures have become progressively tight. As such, the body has compensated for these restrictions thus compromising form and function. As a result, conditions Seniors may experience could include progressive inactivity, insidious weakness, impaired posture, and balance issues to name a few.

Stretching is not the only management tool, but it will be the one emphasized in this section.

BACK FLEXION STRETCHES

The back muscles do a lot of work keeping us upright, especially when gravity is pulling us forward. They get tired, tight, and painful. Functional problems include difficulty bending forward when dressing as we struggle to put on socks, pants or skirts, or to tie shoes or to pick up objects off the floor.

In the bed stretches section, the single and double knee-to-chest pulls were recommended. The following stretches will give you other options.

Option 1: Face an arm chair or something of the equivalent height. Lean forward and grab hold of the arm rests while maintaining straight elbows. Legs are positioned slightly back as if you want to experience a greater challenge; move them back even farther. Bring the right knee up in the middle in the direction of your nose. *Hold* briefly, return, and repeat.

To incorporate rotation with flexion, bring the right knee toward the left elbow. The advantage of this technique is that the weight of the extremity being raised creates traction or an unloading effect to the lower back joints, which is good. How many you do depends on how each one feels.

Option 2: Stand facing up a staircase and far to one side so your shoulder can touch the wall or railing for balance. Place your right foot on the edge of the second step and lean into the knee. *Hold* thirty seconds. This may be performed in many locations as long as your foot prop is stationary and your stance leg is stable.

LOWER BACK ARCH

This is a postural exercise addressed earlier. But, in functional terms, you have been sitting, and, upon standing, you feel stiff and are having difficulty getting fully upright. You are getting a stooped posture and are having a tendency to lose your balance in the forward direction.

Place your hands on your back over where your hip pockets would be. Lean back slightly and arch your back. Do not look up. *Hold* and slowly return.

SIDE BEND OR TORSO STRETCH

Tilting the torso from side to side is a function taking place mostly in the mid and mid back to upper back region. Progressive difficulties may be experienced when reaching overhead, such as putting your arm in a piece of clothing and when you're sitting and leaning over to one side to pick up something.

Option 1: Sit straight in a chair with no arm rests. With your arms outstretched to the sides, bend to one side, *hold* then slowly bend the other and *hold.*

Option 2: Stand straight with feet shoulder width apart, knees slightly bent, and the right hand on your right hip to stabilize the pelvis. Lift the left arm and hand over your head. Motion is isolated in the torso as you side bend toward the right. You may do several stretches to one side in succession or alternate, but regardless, maintain a slight *hold* at the end of each bend as comfort permits. *No jerking!*

Hip flexor stretches. This was another muscle group identified in the postural chapter. Functionally, you may relate hip flexor tightness to having difficulty standing upright, especially at the hips. Your forward tilt gives the appearance that you are "walking into the wind." There may be a tendency to lose your balance in the forward direction, and when walking, your strides are becoming shorter and quicker. All this is not good for balance.

Option 1: Stand with the left foot and leg ahead and knee bent. The right leg is behind, knee straight, and with the weight on the toes which are pointing directly forward. Place your right hand on your right hip pocket area and slowly lunge, keeping upright the entire time with your trunk.

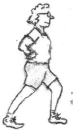

The pulling sensation should be felt in front of the right hip. *Hold* at the end range. For balance measures, this can be done with a shoulder touching a wall, or recruit a spotter.

Option 2: Kneel on the floor with a pillow under your right knee for padding. Position the left leg so the thigh is parallel to the floor and the knee is bent to a 90° angle.

Place your right hand on your right hip pocket and slowly lean backward while maintaining pressure with your right hand.

QUAD STRETCH

The quads are short for quadriceps, a four muscle group on the front of the thigh. Little, if any, thought is given to these muscles unless you have had knee surgery. You find you are having difficulty standing from a sitting position or that stair climbing is progressively more challenging.

Rehabilitation of the quads, like other muscles, takes a three-fold approach—stretching, strengthening, and conditioning. How to mesh these components will be covered later.

As a point of warning, do not attempt to do quad stretches if any of the following situations apply.

You have had or are about to have knee surgery and haven't first gotten medical approval.

You have an arthritic knee or are restricted in knee flexion (bending).

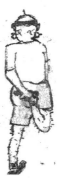

You can't stand on one leg even when holding on for balance. Hold on to something that doesn't move and that will permit you to stand fully upright.

While holding for balance with the left hand, grab the left ankle from behind with your right hand. Pull the left ankle gently toward the buttocks and stand tall. *Hold* and slowly release the tension, but you may want to keep hold of the ankle and do several stretches before stretching the right quad.

CALF STRETCHES

You may see these referred to as heel cord stretches, but, in reality, the heel cords (Achilles tendons) have little if any capacity to stretch. The heel cords are tendons that attach the calf muscles to the heel bones. When doing calf stretches, if you don't feel "pulling" sensations in the calf, reevaluate your form and consider the possibility that you may not need to do them.

Decreased calf flexibility can result from years of wearing high heels, bed or chair confinement after a prolonged recovery process from an injury or illness, or just a progressive sedentary lifestyle.

Functionally tight calf muscles contribute to foot pain, tendencies to catch your toe and trip, fatigue when walking, and difficulty bending.

Position yourself with your arms braced against a wall, one foot several inches behind the other. Bend your front leg, keeping both feet on the floor. Maintain a slow gradual *hold*. For a greater stretch, place the back foot further to the rear.

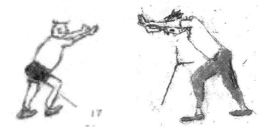

WHAT WAS THAT CHAPTER ALL ABOUT?

Some may view stretching as the nonproductive phase of an exercise program. This is true for those individuals who don't take the time to concentrate on form; for those who don't adhere to the gentle movements and the purposeful *holds* or for those who aren't selective in choosing the stretches that would best address their needs.

Flexibility training assists in joint lubrication and mobility. Stretching is useful in preparing muscles for activity and as a tool to minimize post exercise pain and stiffness. Slow and deliberate stretching enhances coordination and control. Many of the underlying physiological processes linked to balance disorders can be traced back in part to lost flexibility. Discover what requires mobilization, do it, and alter your program as your condition changes.

Chapter 27

TESTING YOUR MUSCLE STRENGTH

In retirement, Seniors often treat their fitness levels as they do their IRAs: "It's okay to draw on the balance, but don't run out before you die!"

Self-strength testing is to identify specific weaknesses so that you can build an exercise program to address those deficiencies.

It is human nature to strengthen what is strong and to ignore what is weak—it's easier that way. Balance issues not only arise from weak muscle groups but also from mismatched strength levels.

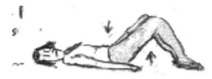

THE ABDOMINAL AND LOWER EXTREMITY MUSCLES

Core Muscle Test. The abdominal muscles are not the only core muscles, but they are a group that is prone to weakness. Lie on your back with bent knees. Tighten your abdominal muscles and try to push your navel toward your spine. The pelvis will rise and the back flattens if you did it correctly. It may take several tries before you figure this one out.

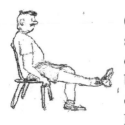

Leg extensions. To assess quadriceps strength (the muscles on the front of the thigh), sit upright or slightly backward. Extend one leg straight in front of you. Holding it for thirty seconds is good for a beginner. Then do the same with the other leg and compare the two. A stopwatch would be good to have for this test.

An ankle test. This is good for both strength and coordination assessment. Lie on your back and cross your legs so the top ankle and foot are free to move in any direction. Then spell out the alphabet using only the ankle, not the whole leg. It doesn't matter if the letters are uppercase or lowercase, printed or written—just be consistent. You should be able to complete the entire alphabet without resting. Repeat with the other ankle.

Toe lifts. Hold on to a counter and attempt to stand on the toes of one foot. Then try the other one. Are the calf muscles weaker in one leg than the other? If you are unable to do this on one foot, try rising to your toes with both feet.

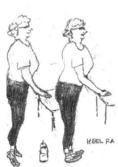

Heel lifts. Do the same exercise as the toe lifts, but raise the toes and stand on your heels.

Foot slaps. If you had difficulty doing toe lifts, you may hear one or both feet slap the ground when the heel touches down. In a few cases, this may only occur when wearing shoes with heels higher than you usually have. Make sure you do this test with little if any heels.

Toe clenching. Take your socks off and check to see if you can really bend the toes on each foot. It's okay if they move as a group.

Getting up from a chair. Slide to the front of the chair, and stand up without using your arms. Make sure your chair doesn't slide out from underneath you. This test assesses several muscle groups but also duplicates an activity we do many times each day.

WHAT WAS THAT CHAPTER ALL ABOUT?

Muscular weakness can be one of several factors contributing to balance problems. When your strength is insufficient to regain your balance, you fall.

Many studies have documented the beneficial effects of strengthening exercises for Seniors. One is to enhance stability and another is to increase bone strength, which also lowers your risk of fracture if you do fall.

Chapter 28

SAFETY IN STRENGTHENING
FOR SENIORS

A DISCERNING MIND

The days of over achieving are over. It's no longer about how much weight you lift for how many reps. The new rules are can you demonstrate control and how to experience fatigue without injury.

Exercise suited to your age status. There are numerous exercise philosophies and even a greater number of exercise machines, each targeting a real or a perceived deficiency in our physical status. It requires wisdom and restraint not to buy and try everything. These promoters are really good!

As you have seen a machine exercise, ask yourself, "How old are you, and did you ever do this before?" Try to imagine if you could ever achieve the speed at which the exercise is demonstrated.

Consider the changes that have occurred in your own physiology over the years versus the challenges these exercise machines place on your systems, and in their abilities to respond. If you are still tempted, review the section on target heart rate and recovery time, plus read on.

THE PRINCIPLE OF STRENGTHENING

This involves overloading the muscles as resistance is applied to a greater degree than would be the case with Anormal" activity. Doing this is not entirely without risk. Proceeding without proper preparation and technique could result in muscle tears, tendon ruptures, and joint trauma, followed by a prolonged recovery process.

Exceeding the speed limit. The key to any successful training process is to maximize muscle loading while simultaneously minimizing musculoskeletal stresses. Both the amount of resistance and the speed of movement must be considered.

The physiological principle that applies here is that the physical stresses are exponentially increased related to the speed of the movement. In other words, double the speed and the forces increase four times. Double that speed and another four times is the stress effect. In this example, a two-pound lift overhead can create eight-to-thirty-pound stresses on the joints, muscles, and connective tissues of the wrist, elbow, and shoulder, just from lifting two pounds faster.

The same principle applies when using elastic bands and tubes, but calculating the exact force is difficult since resistance progressively increases throughout the pull.

However, regardless of the source of the resistance, always keep in mind that fast and jerky movements pose an unnecessary risk and are to be avoided at all times.

PAIN AND EXERCISE

The human body has a built in warning mechanism called pain. Pain alerts you that not all is well. If you are slowly lifting an object, pushing furniture, or bending to reach the floor, you may experience isolated pain, at which time you cease doing what you were about to do. By listening and properly responding to the pain warning, you avoid injury. If you repeat that same activity in a fast manner, you will be unable to stop, thus risking injury.

However, when pursuing a strengthening program, pain can give you insights. For example, if pain is experienced when doing a motion without resistance, then adding weights is not an option. If pain is present immediately after an activity and pain was not there before, reassess your technique.

Experiencing delayed onset pain (twenty-four hours after exercise) can be an indication that you have been too aggressive or need a longer recovery period between strengthening sessions. Too aggressive could include too fast, too many reps, more sets than you should have, or additional resistance was added before you were ready.

Severely deconditioned muscles have been equated to building structures ravished by time and neglect. In order to rebuild, you must first tear them down. There is an element of truth in this concept, but "No pain, no gain" is *not* the message.

What it means is that, in the rebuilding process, pain may be a predictable response from the result of activity but not from injury. Nevertheless, caution must be exercised at all times to minimize the pain response as you progress in an orderly manner with your rebuilding program.

SHOULD I TAKE UP JOGGING?

Frequently during my career as a physical therapist. I had been asked my opinion about numerous physical activities such as jogging. Do you jog? How does it affect you? These were my typical response questions. This also applied to using ankle weights doing step aerobics, as well as participating in many of the vast variety of recreational and physical enhancement programs at our disposal.

There are pros and cons about each potential choice, but my opinion about them is irrelevant to you if you are currently involved in such activity, and it is working. Would I recommend jogging as a first time endeavor to a Senior currently struggling with balance issues? Probably not!

ANKLE WEIGHTS: TO USE OR NOT TO USE

It sounds like a great idea. Strap on a couple ankle weights, go about your business, and before you know it, your legs are strong. You accomplished this without counting reps or going to the gym.

But after a while, the expectation of new-found strength is replaced by the realization that something is wrong. You didn't anticipate that the extra weight at the ankles would put added stress to your feet, ankle, knees, and hips.

The occasional unsteadiness you were coping with seems to be getting more frequent. Your coordination and reactions feel sluggish, and the weights are throwing you off balance. This unfortunate scenario awaits many who choose to use ankle weights.

Every time weight is placed externally onto the body, a physiological chain reaction goes into action to accommodate for the altered forces. Remove the weight and the adaptation process kicks in again. Seniors already struggling with their balance don't need added challenges like this.

Now, it so happens that both Charlie and I have had personal experiences with ankle weights.

Mine occurred in college where I was a sprinter on the track team. I was advised to train with ankle weights. Every day, I put them on and worked on my starts as well as with the sprints. I was feeling strong, conditioned, and confident.

Then came the race. With the ankle weights removed, I exploded from the blocks with absolutely no sense of coordination. It took several weeks of retraining without the weights to regain my old form, which wasn't all that bad to begin with.

As for Charlie, he began to notice that he stumbled once or twice, was getting more unsteady, and his walking was more irregular. Maintaining proper form was getting to be a challenge. Someone suggested exercising with ankle weights. Charlie did gain quad strength, but the trade off was that he was losing his coordination and stability. He quit using the ankle weights.

The Ups And Downs of Stair Climbing

Have you ever heard of the stadium run? It's probably the most grueling and inhumane exercise ever devised.

As part of their conditioning program, athletes run up a flight of stairs, across one section, down a flight of stairs, across, up, across, down, across, up until they circled all or part of the stadium.

The outcomes were not always as anticipated. In addition to falls were muscle pulls, ankle sprains, plantar fasciitis, shin splints, patello-femoral disorders, tendinitis, hip bursitis, and more.

Step aerobics may be a more familiar conditioning technique. Steps of varying heights will change the degree of difficulty and the intensity of the exercises. One step at a time eventually equates to several flights of stairs during the course of one session.

Since this is a graduated program beginning with small steps, I feel it has merit. Besides promoting the strengthening component, step aerobics also enhance the cardiovascular efficiency.

In an effort to burn more calories as well as to enhance our general fitness levels, we often hear that we should take the stairs whenever we can. This bit of advice was included in my weekly diabetes exercise lectures.

Stair climbing for seniors. For most of my professional life, I taught people how to ascend and descend stairs. Postoperative orthopedic patients had to maneuver the stairs with their crutches before they could be discharged. As the years progress, it seems that nothing delays hospital discharges.

We all will be exposed to a flight of stairs at some time or another. Why not practice falling on them as we prepare for that day? There are several reasons why we shouldn't, and they are not necessarily age specific.

First, suppose you are out for a walk. When fatigue sets in, impaired coordination follows and then a risk of falling. You can stop and regroup but it isn't that easy on stairs. I have taught people how to fall on a level surface to minimize injury but never to fall on stairs. I have thought about it, but it's not a risk I am willing to take.

Second, the faster you descend each step, the greater stresses are applied to the feet, ankles, knees, and hip joints and to their corresponding muscles, tendons, and ligaments (exponential forces) than if you descended slowly.

Third, a normal physiological response from a twenty-to-thirty-minute aerobic exercise is fatigue, not to be confused with the abnormal response to climbing a set of stairs causing shortness of breath. This could be a sign of heart or pulmonary distress.

Seniors and stair climbing exercises. The barrier-free movement is eliminating steps and stairs, replacing them with curb cuts, ramps, escalators, and elevators. I have vacationed at a resort where stair climbing is not an option, except for emergency exiting.

Ranch homes and condos are attractive one-level retirement options. Is the general population less fit because stairs have been eliminated from their daily routine? Think about it.

If you are a Senior who finds stairs a challenge, work on the individual components of posture, flexibility, strength, and balance first. Then introduce stair climbing as your condition improves.

Your ability to walk up and down a flight of stairs can also be a way of determining your fitness level. However, always walk the stairs slowly while holding on to the hand rail.

PLYOMETRICS: NOT FOR SENIORS

Many training rooms and physical therapy clinics use plyometrics to develop power in the lower extremities necessary to help athletes jump higher. The athlete stands on a platform then jumps to the floor slightly flexing the knees before springing upward.

I have modified the plyometric concept and used it effectively for nonathletes. For Seniors, I don't advise this exercise without supervision and modification.

WHAT WAS THAT CHAPTER ALL ABOUT?

The theme of this text is of the nature of impaired balance and of corresponding management techniques, but the recurring message is to assure that safety is not compromised by expediency. There are no shortcuts to success when dealing with balance issues.

The exercise mind-set and the physiological responses you had in your 30s no longer apply to you as a Senior. Now, an error in judgment can result in a prolonged and unnecessary recovery process.

Embrace the safety suggestions presented in this chapter as well as throughout the book. In doing so, you will benefit from the wisdom and discernment of those who have gone before.

Chapter 29

GUIDELINES FOR
STRENGTHENING EXERCISES

STRENGTHENING MUSCLES: THE NEXT STEP

Balance issues may not have been a life-long challenge, but, over the past several years, episodes of unsteadiness have crept into your daily routine. These events have gradually become more frequent and perhaps have even contributed to a fall. You have implemented lifestyle changes to protect yourself. However, these have only been reactive measures.

Restoration of upright stability requires an awareness of the underlying causes and contributing factors. The role of posture has been identified, and a case for flexibility training has been presented. The next phase involves strengthening.

DECONDITIONED MUSCLES

How does a muscle used in normal, everyday activities eventually deteriorate to an impaired functional state? A study conducted to address this issue placed electrodes on the quadriceps and recorded electrical responses with individuals walking on level surfaces at a normal pace. The results revealed that the quad activity was minimal.

Charlie tells me he regularly walked with an older friend who did no other exercising. Actually, he says that he started walking with him since his friend always walked faster and further than he did. His friend fell several times, once even breaking his wrist. This statement was in *Consumers Report on Health,* June 2007, "The ankles and thigh muscles of frequent fallers were much weaker than those of similar non-fallers in a recent study of nursing home residents."

What this means to us is that, in order to maintain and to increase strength in any muscle, it needs to be challenged. If a walking program isn't enough to strengthen these muscles, then occasional walks around the house are an insufficient challenge to accomplish either maintenance or increased strength.

As sedentary lifestyles supersede the physical challenges of work and recreation, muscles become deconditioned. Fat infiltrates muscle fibers retarding the quality of the contractions. Their speed of reactions (reflexes), compensating for unexpected influences, slow down. Balance is affected by the inability of the muscles to react and to sustain stability.

UPPER BODY STRENGTHENING

Studies show that those Seniors who increase the strength of their leg muscles will walk with greater ease and enhanced balance. However, no such claims have been made for the arms. This doesn't mean that upper extremity strengthening isn't important, only that it will be given superficial attention in this text.

The beneficial effects of enhanced upper extremity strength are numerous. You are better able to push to get out of a chair, to use a hand rail, to pull yourself up if you should fall, to lift and to carry objects, to use a cane or other walking assists, to open doors, and so forth. Incorporating arm exercises into the rest periods of your leg program is an efficient use of time.

THE REST OF THE STORY: THE IMPORTANCE OF RESTS

So often, too much attention is given to the workout and not enough to the rest period. In reality, rest is the most important component of an exercise program. On the other hand, some people adopt the resting philosophy and ignore the exercise. Exercise and rest, when properly blended, yield optimal results.

How long are rests between strengthening sets? A set is the total number of repetitions performed consecutively. Ideally, the range of reps will be from five to ten when lifting with a ten-second count and returning in five seconds. Fatigue will be experienced as you approach your maximum reps followed by a thirty-second rest period.

During this rest, you may do a mild stretch to the area being strengthened or walk around to keep limber. Regardless, if you don't feel that you have recovered adequately in sixty seconds to continue with another set, your last series was too intense. Your goal is three sets before moving on.

Recovery time. A severely deconditioned muscle will feel the stress of activity with fewer reps and less resistance but will take longer to recover—maybe three to six days. A conditioned muscle will respond well to a ten-rep, three-set exercise routine and may need twenty-four to forty-eight hours to recover. A well-developed muscle will maintain strength with a once-a-week intense workout.

Guidelines for defining recovery times are not necessarily measured in days, but rather by the body's ability to respond to the exercise-induced stresses.

One way is to determine recovery time is how long it takes for the delayed onset pain to go away. Another guide, not related to comfort, is in your ability to equal or to exceed the poundage and reps from your last workout. If you are unable, you haven't recovered.

Never challenge a muscle when it is still in the recovery process. It's okay to stretch but not to strengthen.

Posture principles are ongoing, never needing a day to rest. Balancing and gentle stretching seven days a week can be therapeutic. Recovery time is often a good night's rest. For six days a week, a mix of moderate aerobic and strengthening exercises can be pursued, but, on the seventh day, your body needs a day to recover.

When developing a personal rehabilitation program, take these and other guidelines into consideration. Begin slowly and carefully, even if it means you do too little for a while. Be dedicated to your plan adapting it constantly. This includes your workout routine as well as your recovery times.

THE CORE OF THE PROBLEM

Impaired balance is a problem when the body's orientation in space is lost, and the compensatory mechanism has difficulty finding it. This can happen after a stroke, as a result of injury, with physical changes over time, as well as with many other scenarios. However, the focus at this time must be to identify a deficiency that can be treated and to propose a plan to counteract it.

If this were a math problem, we would be looking for the common denominator, the one deficiency that applies to the majority of balance problems. This is very likely weakness in the core muscles, which directly control trunk mobility and positioning.

Two of these muscle groups are the abdominals and the back extensors. However, the quadriceps, hamstrings, gluteus maximus, and all the other hip muscles are equally important.

When treating a complex condition such as impaired balance, the strengthening program needs to be further expanded since the mechanism involved in retaining and regaining balance must be the union of *all* muscle groups.

If this is so, why not work exclusively on strengthening?

Prior steps. The foundation of every strengthening program must be form. The proper positioning of the extremities can only be achieved when the trunk is optimally aligned.

Therefore, prior to pursuing arm and leg strengthening exercises, you must first develop trunk mobility and control. This means adhering to the posture principles and incorporating the stretching techniques previously presented.

This is really a brilliant concept. Putting forth maximum effort to achieve your best possible posture and faithfully pursuing stretching to promote mobility are both contributing to a process that strengthens the core muscles. By the time you are ready to target the core muscles for strengthening, they already have had a head start.

All strengthening exercises are most efficiently performed with optimal posture, form, and mobility. Demonstrating success in these categories will prepare you well for the balance program, if you are still having balance issues by then.

WHAT WAS THAT CHAPTER ALL ABOUT?

Muscles become deconditioned when one leads a sedentary life. Strengthening the upper body muscles is helpful, but for the unsteady, the lower body muscles must be strengthened. A strengthening program needs rest and recovery periods. Most important it should be preceded by posture and flexibility exercises to achieve proper form.

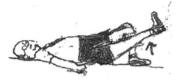

Chapter 30

STRENGTHENING EXERCISES

ABDOMINAL STRENGTHENING

Pelvic tilt. Lie supine with knees bent. Tighten your abdominal muscles. This pushes your belly button toward the spine. The arch in your back flattens.

Lower abdominals. Lie supine with knees bent. Keep one knee bent and extend the opposite leg. Then slowly lower it to the ground. Bend it and repeat alternately.

Variation: Put cuff weights on the ankles.

Crunches. Lie supine with knees bent and arms to the sides. Begin by doing a pelvic tilt by tightening the abdominals so that you feel your shoulders lifting or less pressure on your shoulder blades.

Caution: Do not bend your head and neck forward.

Variation: Increase the difficulty by placing your hands on your abdomen or cross your arms at the chest.

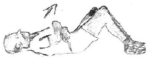

Obliques variation: Same as the crunch except extend one arm to the opposite knee.

Note: There is no need to go any farther than to feel the contraction of the abdominals. Always move slowly and never put your hands behind your neck.

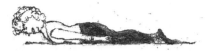

BACK EXTENSOR STRENGTHENING

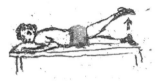

Back hyperextensions. Lie prone with one or two pillows under your waist. With arms at your sides, slowly lift your upper body. A three-second hold would be plenty long for this exercise. It is helpful to have someone hold the feet and legs.

Leg extensions. Lie prone on a bed with your hips at the edge and legs hanging down. Extend one leg to the rear. Then alternate right and left.

Variation: See SLR extension to follow.

STRAIGHT LEG RAISES (SLR)

Flexion. Lie supine with the left knee bent and foot flat. Raise the extended right leg three inches and *hold* up to seconds. Slowly return to the rest position and repeat.

Abduction. Lie on your right side with the right leg bent and the left leg extended (straight). Raise the left leg up six inches. Do not roll your leg outward when lifting.

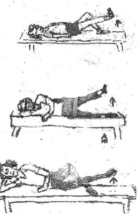

Extension. Lie prone, raise the extended right leg a few inches. Do not roll your leg outward when lifting. Okay to alternate right and left legs.

Adduction. Lie on your right side with the right leg extended. Bend the left knee and place the left foot flat in front of the right leg. Raise the right leg up but don't be concerned about how far.

QUADRICEPS (QUADS)

Quad sets. Lie supine with one leg straight. Tighten the thigh muscles on the straight leg pushing that knee down.

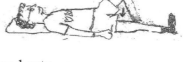

Variation: Precede SLR flexion with quad sets.

Supine. Lie supine with a tightly rolled towel under the knees. Alternately straighten one leg at a time. Don't forget to *hold* the fully extended position at least ten seconds and use cuff weights as you advance.

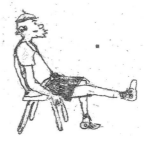

Sitting extension. Sit leaning slightly backward and extend one leg at a time. It's okay to alternate.

Variation: If you feel crunching in your knee caps, use this variation. Support your feet on a small foot stool or a large pillow before doing the extensions.

Variation: For a variety, hold your legs slightly rolled inward, outward, or straight when doing an extension.

SQUATS

There are many excellent strengthening exercises, but few have the functional carry over that squatting has. Squats target the quads, hamstrings, and buttock muscles that are incorporated in activities like stair climbing, sitting, standing, walking on levels and inclines, and lifting.

The squatting variations have different degrees of difficulty. Your ability to do any of them, however, may depend on your current fitness level and/or the existence of physical problems. Never do a squat that puts you in a position of vulnerability for falling or knee irritation.

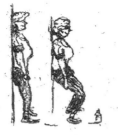

Wall slides. Stand with your back against a wall, feet shoulder width and about a foot away from the wall. Slowly sink down to a 45° angle maintaining wall contact with your back. Work up to a ten second hold before standing. If you are a skier, sixty seconds at 90° is your goal.

Chair squats. Back up to an arm chair that is secured from moving. Reach back for the chair arms and begin to sit; however, stop before you do and stand back up. If your legs give out or you lose your balance, the worst that can happen is that you sit down.

Unassisted squats. These are by far the most challenging of all the squats. You must have normal ankle mobility, which means no calf tightness. Also, don't attempt these until you have mastered the wall slides and chair squats.

These squats are done standing with the knees slightly bent and feet shoulder width apart. Hands are held out straight or holding on to something especially when first attempting them. Slowly bend to 45° and return. Remember, no bouncing; go easy if you have "bad" knees, and keep your back straight. On the other hand, to make it harder, go slower, not deeper.

Lunges. Lunges incorporate the principles of balance, stretching, and strengthening Hold on to a counter top for balance assistance. The starting position has the right leg in front and the left foot to the rear.

Keep your back upright and slowly shift your weight forward onto a bending right knee. At the same time, the left knee remains straight. The heel of the rear foot may slightly come off the floor.

You should feel a pulling sensation in front of the right hip, which is a stretch of the hip flexors. The strengthening effect is in the left quad. Unlike squats, a lunge can be used to strengthen one quad, which comes in handy if the other knee is unable to go into a squatting position.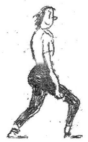

Hip flexors. Hip flexors initiate the forward motion of the hind leg when walking and lifts the lower extremity when stepping. Weakness can contribute to a shuffling gait pattern, which can result in catching a toe.

Other problems including weak hip flexors include toe catching, difficulty stepping over objects, and walking up stairs.

Sitting strengthening. Sitting in a kitchen chair with both feet flat on the floor, lift one knee upward. It's okay to alternate leg lifts. Lifts are slow with a *hold* at the top. It is not a marching motion.

Hamstrings. Assume the same starting position as with standing hip flexor strengthening. Keep your thighs together and bend the right leg so your heel rises behind you. The right calf should be parallel to the floor at the end of the lift.

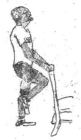

Standing strengthening. Do not attempt to do this if the standing leg is too weak to support your weight. Hold on to a counter top or chair, keep your back straight, and raise a knee forward and upward.

ANKLES

Heel raise. Stand near a counter and hold on. Rise up on your toes as far as you can. Lower and then rock back on your heels. *Rest* and slowly repeat.

Toe raise. Stand near a counter and hold on. Lift up your toes keeping legs straight. Then lower your toes until your feet are once again flat on the floor. *Rest* and slowly repeat.

Heel walking. Walk near a counter or wall. With your legs straight, take short steps putting weight only on your heels.

Heel raise: sitting. While sitting, rise up on your toes.

Toe taps: sitting.

216

Heel raises and toe taps. Combine the last two exercises while in the comfort of your easy chair. Alternate up and down, left and right. While sitting, raise your toes up keeping your heels on the floor.

TOES

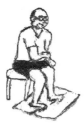

Toe scrunch. Sit with your shoes and socks off. Place two towels on the floor. Keep your feet shoulder width apart and attempt to grasp as much of the towel as you can with your toes and pull it toward you. Try one foot at a time until you learn the exercise.

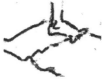

Toe pickups. Scatter twenty marbles on the rug. Pick them up with your toes and put them in a bowl. Make sure that you count the marbles when you are done so that there are none left on the floor.

WHAT WAS THAT CHAPTER ALL ABOUT?

It takes work to become a Senior, and. once we have arrived, it is like many other accomplishments. We dwell on the achievement rather than on the process and on the effort necessary to get there. Gradually, we experience muscular strength deficiencies and loss of bone density. As balance issues kick in, activity is further curtailed.

Reversing the downward trend is not only possible, but it is also a realistic goal, but it takes work. Strengthening is yet another instrument for your rehabilitation tool box.

Chapter 31

GUIDELINES FOR BALANCE

HOW MANY REPETITIONS OF EACH EXERCISE?

No particular number of reps. Two limiting factors are your ability to maintain focus and your fatigue factor. A good repetition guideline is to stop when the results of your efforts deteriorate.

WHEN IS THE LEAST FAVORABLE TIME TO WORK ON BALANCE?

Reflect back when you first began to have balance issues. Upon first rising in the morning, your balance wasn't that great. Bedroom furniture was handy to hold on to as you made your way to the bathroom. Then came the challenge of standing on one leg to put on a sock or of slipping your foot into a piece of clothing. Everything that contributed to impaired balance then is even more pertinent today.

THE PHYSIOLOGICAL ISSUES AFFECTING BALANCE

On getting up. Your eyes aren't ready to focus. The pupils remain dilated for a while making them sensitive to light, thus the tendency to squint. You will notice a dramatic improvement in your ability to balance with your eyes open versus closed.

Sleeping and being relatively inactive for eight hours takes weight off our joints with little movement occurring throughout the body. This permits the infusion of water resulting in morning stiffness.

Stretching in bed will improve joint mobility to a degree, but standing and moving about forces excess fluids from the weight-bearing joints and the spine. As such, practicing balance in the presence of stiff and possibly more painful joints could be counterproductive.

Along the same line, the muscles and related reflexes are sluggish upon awakening. Challenging them; to react appropriately to balance exercises before they have a chance to "wake up" and "warm up" puts them at a disadvantage.

Even though we sleep, the bodily functions continue to draw upon blood sugars for energy. Normally, this would have little if any impact on balance exercises. However, if you are a diabetic or are prone to having low blood sugar, your balance, vision, and comfort could be affected.

Loss of balance when your feet first hit the floor, after lying down, may be your motivation for pursuing this program. If this is when your balance is most challenged, it makes sense to practice when you most need it.

However, what may be occurring is orthostatic hypotension. The blood rushes from the head, and your blood pressure drops and maybe you along with it. It's not a good idea to stand without sitting for a moment while your circulation adapts to the new position.

The worst times throughout the day. The worst time to do balance exercises is just before any meal when your blood sugar may be low.

When is the best time to do balance exercises? Ideally, balance exercises are most successfully performed when you are well rested and after you have eaten. It's further enhanced once you have stretched, had a chance to be on your feet a while, and when you are not rushed. This is an excellent opportunity to get acquainted with new balancing techniques.

How long should a balance position be held? Confidently holding a balance position for thirty seconds is sufficiently long enough to consider progressing to the variations. However, don't become discouraged by slow progress since you are relearning a motor skill. Holding a position greater than thirty seconds is also acceptable.

Additional insights concerning balance exercises. Go ahead and familiarize yourself with the balance exercises in your ideal environment. Then use your imagination on how to make the exercise more difficult, like the introduction of distractions.

Reflect on the circumstances when your balance is most challenged, and it may not be in the confines of your home.

WHAT WAS THAT CHAPTER ALL ABOUT?

This chapter answers questions frequently asked and gives specific guidelines for doing balance exercises.

Chapter 32

BALANCE EXERCISES

DOUBLE-LEG STANCE

A basic exercise. Stand in the middle of a door frame with equal weight on both feet. Let go with the hands. This can also be done standing at a sink or anywhere that you can grab hold of if needed.

Variations:
1. Close your eyes.
2. Hold your arms still but away from your sides.
3. Do arm circles with eyes open then closed.

SINGLE LEG STANCE

A basic exercise. Stand in the middle of a door frame lightly touching the frame. Slowly lift one leg and *hold*. Then repeat with the opposite leg.

Variations:
1. Do not hold on.
2. Close your eyes.
3. Hold your arms still but away from the body at first with the eyes open then closed.

HIP CIRCLES

Stand on both feet at a counter touching with light finger pressure without moving your shoulders or your feet. Make circles with your hips. Start with small circles and gradually make larger ones. Go clockwise then counter clockwise.

Variation: Repeat the same exercise with your eyes closed and your feet closer together.

Weight shift. Stand with your feet shoulder length apart. Slowly shift your weight from one foot to the other. Never lose contact with the floor. Touch the counter top if needed.

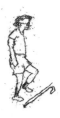

March in place. This is better done facing a corner or in a doorway rather than at a counter because you won't hit your knees. Stand in place and lift your right knee toward your chest then the left knee. A light touch may be required at first.

Variations:
1. Lift the knees higher as comfort and safety permit.
2. Incorporate arm swings—Right knee up, and the left arm bends at the elbow and comes forward. Repeat with the left knee and right arm.

TOE TAPS

This is best done standing sideways to a counter. Touch or hold on to the counter with your left hand and stand on your left leg.

Then the fun and your imagination begin. Tap the right toe underneath you, in front, behind, out to the side, or in any combination of your choice. Don't forget to turn around and tap the opposite foot.

Variations:
1. Vary both the pattern and the speed of the tapping.
2. You may even try to do leg circles in both directions.

SIDE STEPPING

Hold on to the counter if you need to. Begin with your legs together, and then take a step to the right side with your right leg. Bring your left leg to meet the right one. Do five and then five side steps to the left.

Variations:
1. Vary the speed keeping in mind that the slower you step, the harder it is to do.
2. Wean your way from touching as you feel safer.

THE GRAPEVINE (CROSSOVER-WALKING)

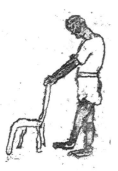

Do this facing the kitchen counter. Step to the side with your right foot then cross in front with the left then to the side with the right and behind with the left. When you run out of room, go the other directions.

HEEL-TO-TOE WALK

Find a line in the carpet pattern; put a chalk line on the basement floor, or use a smooth, straight crack line in a tiled floor. Walk along this straight line trying to hit the line alternately with each heel. Use your hand for support when necessary. A narrow hallway that would allow you to use both walls is ideal.

Variations:
1. Do on a treadmill while at a slow speed and when you are holding on.
2. A less difficult variation is to use the same line but walk heel to toe on either side of it. Your stance may be wide at first and then narrower as you improve.

3. When you can walk heel to toe in a straight line without holding on and still keep your balance, you are now ready for the Senior Balance Beam Competition.

BALANCE TRAINING EQUIPMENT

Balance training can be effectively pursued without equipment, but there are devices that further challenge the balance mechanism. I have used them in my clinic to increase flexibility, for strengthening as well as to enhance balance.

The exercise equipment may seem easy enough to use, but in a do-it-yourself project, it isn't worth the risk. Seek out professional insight as to which devices best suit your needs, guidance on how to safely and effectively use each one, and instruction on constructing the ones that can be built.

Osteoballs. These are excellent for core strengthening and balance training. They usually come with a foot or hand pump for inflation and an instructional booklet.

Wobble boards. These consist of a round platform about sixteen inches across. Attached to the bottom is a circular pivoting device about the size of a baseball. The plan is to stand on this board, rock backward and forward, side to side, and to do circles clockwise and counterclockwise.

Foam squares. A piece of 4' x 4' foam can be purchased at fabric stores. The softness and thick consistency of the foam increases the degree of difficulty. This flexible surface is also an excellent choice to practice with your bare feet. Since the foam is not rigid, the toes, feet, ankles, and hips are all incorporated in adapting to the body's changing positions to maintain balance. Try some of the in-place balance exercises on the foam. Either with or without shoes, the foam has tremendous carryover benefits to balancing in the "real world."

Unstable surfaces. Weeble boards, foam squares, rubber exercise domes, pillows, and other devices create challenges to your balance, proprioception, and stability.

Prerequisites for incorporating unstable surfaces into your training program are:

1. You are able to incorporate correct posture.
2. You have developed sufficient flexibility and strength.
3. You have demonstrated success in the basic balancing techniques.
4. You are able to hold on to a stable support in good posture when attempting these activities.

WHAT WAS THAT CHAPTER ALL ABOUT?

Balance is a motor skill that is externally influenced by environmental occurrences and internally by its interdependency on the influences of other body systems. The prognosis for recovering balance skills may depend on the identification and management of what caused the deterioration in the first place.

However, one thing is for sure, do nothing but wait, and balance skills will get worse.

Organization of a balance program includes dedicating a time each day to work on specific skills. Keep accurate records and advance in the degree of difficulty when success has been achieved at the more elementary levels.

There also may be a progression to where you practice during the times of the day least favorable for balance. This will further challenge your ability to adapt to more difficult circumstances in daily living.

The remaining aspect of training is to incorporate balance principles in your daily activities. Take frequent breaks from sitting to stretch to stand and to restore proper, upright posture. Balance while watching the evening news, when doing dishes, as you walk about, etc. As with any motor skill, improvement depends on practice—perfect practice that is!

Chapter 33

WALKING

Walking is the functional activity we use most until the day arrives when we struggle to maintain our balance. Then it becomes the most feared.

The preceding chapters have presented a logical explanation as to the contributing factors of progressive inactivity, deviated postures, decreased mobility, and strength loss to impaired balance. As such, it is unrealistic to expect that stability in walking can be regained strictly by walking more.

The benefits of a walking program are well documented, but before it can be considered as aerobic conditioning, Seniors must first demonstrate that they are able to walk safely as they pursue their activities of daily living.

This chapter will further explore the subject of balance with emphasis on the restoration of a safe and efficient ability to ambulate. Accomplishment of this will dictate the consideration of using walking as a conditioning tool as well.

WALKING AS YOUR SOLE EXERCISE

As noted earlier, Charlie had a friend who could walk faster and farther than he could, yet he fell several times, once even breaking his wrist. This is because walking does not strengthen the quadriceps.

When you feel you are about to fall, in order to stay upright, the ankle and thigh muscles reflexively prevent it or you stumble forward.

It is worth repeating, the statement was in the *Consumers Report on Health*, June 2007: "The ankles and thigh muscles of frequent fallers were much weaker than those of similar non-fallers in a recent study of nursing home residents."

This doesn't mean unsteady Seniors should give up walking. It is a good all-around exercise. But they should not make it their sole exercise.

CREATING A SAFE ENVIRONMENT FOR YOUR WALKING

As we age, there is no such thing as "status quo." You know this; otherwise, why would you be reading this text now? Our inability to recognize these changes and to adjust accordingly can have dire consequences.

Remember, when you are coping with balance issues of any kind, safety is a major concern. One fall can be the determining factor between independence and confinement.

As a physical therapist, I have been impressed by how creative individuals are when it comes to injuring themselves. It's not surprising that, in some way, most or even all of these calamities could have been avoided.

The following is a compilation of situations with negative ramifications. Do you relate to any of them? They are neither isolated nor theoretical events, and they are not age specific.

They come from the histories of my patients. Charlie has listed some of them in his chapters, but it won't hurt to repeat them for emphasis.

Studies have shown that a person is more likely to be injured in and around his/her home than anywhere else. Retired Seniors generally spend more time in their homes than do those working outside the home. The solution is *not* to move but rather to make the home a safer place in which to live.

Do you have a tendency to lose your balance when looking down because you're afraid that you may trip over the clutter on the stairs and floors or because you have an obstacle course in the basement, garage, or on the lawn?

If looking up makes you dizzy, don't paint the ceiling or stand outside and gaze at the sky. In many situations, just looking up as you retrieve something off the top shelf may be sufficiently long enough to trigger an episode.

If you are unsteady on the stairs, why not free up a hand to hold on to the railing; fix the railing, or what about having a railing installed?

You have noticed that it is becoming harder to pick up your feet, and others have commented on your shuffle. Why not get rid of the throw rugs before they throw you?

If maneuvering safely in the bathroom is a challenge, have grab bars professionally installed. It may seem like an easy-enough home project until you realize someday that its ability to prevent you from falling will depend upon how secure it is.

You know that a dark environment disrupts your balance, but you prefer to sleep in a dark room rather than adjust to a night light. Did you know there are devices that permit you to turn on the room light from your bed?

If you are the do-it-yourself type and think that climbing the ladder to clean out the gutters or shoveling snow off the porch roof is saving you money, you may be amazed to find out how expensive a fall can be.

WALKING THE DOG

Are you a little unstable when you're walking the dog, or should I say when the dog is walking you?

If you have difficulty regaining your balance when "tripped up," have you forgotten that your pet's favorite way to get attention is to hang around your feet? Have you considered the leash that insidiously snakes around your ankles?

SKIPPING BREAKFAST

Your blood sugar is consistently low every morning but you continue to put off breakfast. Perhaps you're going to a brunch in a couple hours and don't want to ruin your appetite. You don't feel like exercising after you eat, so you do it right after you get up. You're late and will grab a bite later.

MEDICATIONS

Are you aware that many medications blunt your senses and your reaction time? Always find out the side effects of each new medication, and then see how you react to it. Your unsteadiness and dizziness may be induced by a medication. Many of them say don't drive after taking them, but few warn you not to walk!

YOUR NORMAL WALK

I once critiqued a very interesting pattern of ambulation; after which time, my patient responded, "Well, this is my 'normal' walk." Not much thought went into the quality of the movements as long as they got him where he was going.

An abnormal walking style is more than an issue of aesthetics. It can be inefficient and fatiguing as well as unsafe. Even if you perceive that your walking is not normal, you may still not know how to fix it, even if you wanted to.

Walking was once simplistically described only as putting one foot ahead of the other. In reality, it is balancing on one leg and then the other.

For this reason, those leg strengtheners and one-legged balance exercises make a lot of sense. To go a step further, I will break down the phases that each leg goes through in a stride.

THE CYCLE IN NORMAL WALKING

Would you know a "normal" walk if you saw one? After I describe one in detail, you will be amazed on how few perfect gaits there are out there. Here are the elements.

Stance. This is when all of your weight is on one leg. It begins when the heel touches and ends when the toe comes off the ground.

Swing phase. As the foot leaves the surface, it goes into the swing phase. The knee bends, and the ankle flexes upward to prevent tripping as the leg passes under. The knee extends as the heel prepares to strike the ground. During the entire swing phase, the opposite leg is in stance phase.

Heel strike. The heel hits the pavement, first followed by the rest of the foot, which will maintain surface contact until just before push off.

Push off. The ball of your foot, the toes, and primarily the big toe pushes from behind giving you forward momentum. This propulsion also advances the body's center of gravity.

A coordinated pattern occurs when the heel strike of one foot is simultaneous with the push off of the other foot. A normal stride is when the heel lands about one to one and a half shoe lengths ahead of the other foot. The foot is *slightly* turned out during stance, which enhances balance and provides for a more efficient push off.

Individuals struggling with balance tend to walk faster to minimize the one-legged stance phase but, in doing so, fall more often. Slow walking is a specialized skill requiring enhanced balancing abilities.

Arm swings. These are often a neglected but necessary element of a normal walk. They assist with the rhythm of the gait and act as a balance check. As one arm swings forward, the opposite arm is extending backward.

Each arm movement goes in the same direction and moves at the same speed as does the opposite leg. This opposing action twists the trunk and contributes to trunk mobility. Are you having difficulty swinging the arms? Do more trunk stretches.

Arm swings also contribute to an efficient and balanced stride. The opposite and equal arm movements are just as important as those in the legs.

Achieving a normal walk exclusively through an awareness of the mechanics of a step is helpful but unlikely. The following chapter will explore several abnormal walking styles, the contributing biomechanical factors, and correction suggestions.

WALKING WITH A CANE

Canes have been used as a fashion statement, for a support device, and as a balance aid. Regardless of why you utilize one, the same rule applies—do not alter the arm swing of the normal gait just because you are holding on to a cane.

If one leg is weak, put the cane in the opposite hand; advance the cane as the opposite leg swings, and maintain contact with the walking surface when the affected leg is in stance.

As you approach a set of stairs, the cane can be switched to permit you to hold the railing. Since arm swings are not a factor when on stairs, the cane remains on the step of the affected leg. Resist the urge to carry the cane. Hold the railing with one hand, and use the cane with the other.

If balance is a concern with no particular, one-leg problem, hold the cane in your non-dominant hand. This frees the dominant one to function. However, it may be switched at any time, but, at all times, adhere to the arm swing rule.

There is a lot of resistance in the area of using a cane in the opposite hand when providing support. The argument is that the cane should be held on the same side and act like an artificial leg, so to speak.

The first problem with this is that the opposite arm swing is no longer effective as a balance check. Second, if the cane should slip, most of all your weight is placed on the affected leg. Third, when it comes time to ditch the cane, you have developed a "hitch" in your walk by practicing an abnormal walking pattern.

Chester in "Gunsmoke" and House both used a cane in the wrong hand. House knew it, Chester didn't.

If you are self-conscious about using a cane, get a fancy one and make a fashion statement.

Walking With a Walker

Walkers are four-legged support devices that are lifted, slid, or rolled and slid. Note that a grocery cart is a kind of temporary walker.

For the purpose of this text, I point out that, regardless of the technique used, they all encourage a forward lean, rounded back and shoulder positions, and a forward head. Walkers eliminate arm swing and encourage short steps and a shuffle gait.

To counteract the abnormal positional stresses induced by walker use, put more effort into your postural routines and resting posture positions. If a walker is used only for balance awareness, it is possible to stand erect and walk, however, still with no arm swing,

USING HAND WEIGHTS

These can be effectively incorporated into a walking program, providing you don't have heart disease, high blood pressure, or joint problems. If you do, get medical clearance before beginning.

If using hand weights diverts your attention from what your legs are supposed to be doing, don't use them. If hand weights throw you off balance when walking, wait until you are more stable before trying them. Never use hand weights when walking on stairs or on a treadmill! Hold on to the railings.

If you are interested in using hand weights, here are the guidelines. Initially use one pound weights and gradually work up to three pounds, providing you are able to maintain control of them at all times.

Complement the weight movements with the pace of your walk. This is for balance control. Also, as your confidence builds, incorporate a variety of directional movements such as elbow flexing, punching, or to the sides, shrugging, etc. The changes in direction will minimize the chance of fatigue or of sustaining a repetitive stress injury.

WALKING FOR EXERCISE

Now that the principles of posture, stretching and strengthening plus the mechanics of walking have been addressed, it may be time to consider introducing an aerobic activity into your program.

Walking is a natural choice because you already do it; the expense can be minimal, and the carryover effect is outstanding (gait strengthening in physical therapy terms).

BENEFITS OF WALKING

There are many negative aspects of obesity, but bone density doesn't seem to be one. The excessive weight strengthens the bones in the lower extremities. However, in an effort to reduce, many choose to decrease what they eat without regard to nutrition. As the weight comes off, the bone density progressively decreases.

A twelve-year study involving sixty-one thousand Senior women found that those who took walks of up to four hours a week had 41 percent fewer hip fractures. Even those who walked an hour once a week had 6 percent fewer hip fractures.

Increasing the pace of the walk further reduces the incidence of hip fractures, but don't walk any faster than your comfort levels allow.

Are you interested in preventing the growth of fat around the gut? A study at Duke University Medical Center found that if you walk eleven miles a week (which is quite a bit), you can accomplish this.

Balancing exercises improve our walking, but what about the other way around? A study of 161 Seniors, sixty-five and over, conducted by the University of Michigan, showed that after a ten-week walking program, their balance and mobility improved more than in the group that participated only in Tai Chi.

Improvement was noted in the increased stride and faster walking pace. The differential advantage, according to researchers, was the importance of the movement involved in walking versus Tai Chi.

WALKING POSTURE

By now, this should be review. Stand tall as you walk with your arms hanging relaxed at your sides being free to swing. Do not bend over and look at the ground. Avoid jutting the head forward since this puts a strain on the neck and disrupts blood flow that can create dizziness.

Focus your eyes on the horizon and tilt your head down slightly to permit you to gaze to fifteen to twenty feet ahead. This should permit you to see where you will be stepping next. Reach with each step so that the heel hits first. This will prevent you from catching your toe in a crack in the walk.

PLANNING YOUR WALK

For a walking program to be effective, it should be pursued every day. Walking outside is inexpensive and gets us fresh air. You get to know your neighbors as well as their pets. Your neighbors will notice, and you may be a source of motivation for them to get out and walk as well.

There are only a few days when the elements may prevent you from walking. One authority says not to walk when the winds are over 15 mph. Check the weather first or how fast the debris is blowing down the street.

Other deterrents are electrical storms and icy/snowy conditions. You can adjust for a gentle rain, cold weather, and excessive heat. If you don't think this can be done, don't tell me; tell the 80+-year-old lady who lived in my neighborhood and was an inspiration by her dedication.

Before beginning your program, map out a course and then measure the distance with your car. If you think you can't make it back, have someone follow in a car. Take note of landmarks and shorter distances along the way as you are getting into your distance goal. Good advice is to stick with your same route each day and to inform someone of your routine.

Some walking experts recommend you begin with a slow warm up of five minutes of walking and end with a similar time of slow down. I prefer doing this as opposed to going through a pre-walking stretching routine. Stretching after a "power walk" is advisable.

A good progression for the beginner is to start walking for fifteen minutes and gradually work up to an hour. Another measurement of progression is how fast you are walking. Progress is covering the same distance in less time.

Keeping a walking diary can be a good motivator. Also note how often you stopped to talk. If you miss walking more than three days in a row, you should start back slowly.

Nordic Walking

The Scandinavians have come up with a new walking exercise that causes you to burn 40 percent more energy than ordinary walking. It's done with two aluminum or titanium poles with plastic hand grips and spear tips with discs called paws, which keep you from sinking too far into mud.

The poles are just like those that skiers use except that the spear ends have a special retractable tip that also allows you to walk on hard surfaces such as concrete. The poles cost between seventy and two hundred dollars a pair. The theory is that the arms physically assist with the walking. This reduces knee stress.

Trying this it with two canes may result is your walking faster and may feel like less work, but that's deceiving. It will strengthen your upper body muscles and is a balance aid.

WALKING ON THE BEACH

It is not unusual for Seniors to migrate to the beaches both for their residences and vacations. Is walking on the beach a good or bad idea? The answer is: it depends.

Why should I avoid beach walking? Considering the theme of this text, we must first address the question: What effect does the beach environment have on balance? Do the self tests determine how good or how bad your balance is when standing still, moving, or exposed to external forces like wind?

If you are unable to stand on one leg on your kitchen floor without tipping over, *no beach*.

If any uneven surface throws you off balance, *no beach*.

If you are easily distracted which causes you to lose your balance, *no beach*.

If your equilibrium is affected by rolling waves, bright sunshine (lights), and/or winds, *no beach*.

There are probably more variables and obstacles on a beach than anywhere else you would choose to practice walking. Shells, rocks, driftwood, children's toys, and liter on top of the sand and under the surface lying in wait for the unsuspecting walker. (Charlie stepped on a buried fish bone and got an infected foot.)

Beaches are often sloped, and if walking with one foot higher than the other makes it difficult to remain upright, *no beach*.

How can beach walking be beneficial? Walking in sand utilizes the overtraining principle. If you can do this, then walking on predictable, firm surfaces will be no problem. Use those variable beach conditions to your advantage.

The uneven surfaces, the slopes, the sea breezes and the looseness of the sand will challenge your core and leg muscles as they kick in as balance checks and propulsion.

Foot and toe exercises were addressed in the strengthening section. Now, consider the workout those tiny foot joints and muscles get as they maneuver around thousands of grains of sand.

Don't be surprised if you are unable to walk as far or as fast on a beach than on dry land. This type of walking is fatiguing, and your feet may be the body part that needs the longest time to recover.

It's a good idea not to walk in the heat of the day. If you can find a shady spot, just stand or sit and "work" the sand with your toes and feet. If the sand is soft, hold on to a friend and practice balancing. You'll notice a big difference compared to doing them at home in front of the sink.

Beach hardness. I don't advise walking in sand where your feet sink into it. It's too fatiguing and not much fun, plus you won't get too far.

However, there are some places like Daytona Beach, which is hard enough to drive a car on, and they do. That surface is too hard on the feet to walk barefoot, and sandals don't give your feet adequate support. Shoes work well.

If you are not at risk for falling, you may consider taking in a beach walk in the cool of the day. You may like it.

WALKING SHOES

A successful walking program is only as effective as the selection of the proper footwear. What is comfortable around the house or for everyday activities may not be appropriate on a thirty-minute walk repeated day after day. The most comfortable shoes are often the broken-in and broken-down variety.

Consider the numerous foot ailments and the wide variety of shoes. The consumer must seek professional assistance. The days of buying a pair of all-purpose "tennis shoes" is long gone. Self-help shoe store bargains are disasters waiting to happen, but you can find a deal if you know what to look for.

Purchase a walking shoe from a retailer with specialized shoes and technicians. Proper shoes provide support, assist in balance, effectively distribute pressure, and act as shock absorbers.

Two final pieces of walking advice: Never buy used shoes, and always drink plenty of water.

WHAT WAS THAT CHAPTER ALL ABOUT?

Just like balance, walking is a motor skill, and we can train to improve its aesthetics, efficiency, and power. A walking style that looks good will also lessen the risk of tripping. An efficient walk enhances endurance sufficiently to incorporate walking into more daily activities as well as to expand your recreational options.

A confident and secure walk will make it possible to consider walking as an aerobic conditioning tool. The benefits at this level of intensity include the enhancement of systemic circulation, trunk mobility, core and extremity strengthening, and respiration. Aerobics also release endorphins and enkephalins into the bloodstream. These are the natural pain relievers that also make us feel good.

As valuable as walking is, it is one of the first things we shy away from when balance is compromised. In reality, walking is the tool needed to restore balance.

CHAPTER 34

CORRECTING WALKING PROBLEMS

Deviations from the "normal" are compensatory reactions to problems. Recognizing the distinctive features of each abnormal gait often dictates the plan of correction.

Individuals dealing with balance problems and irreversible structural changes within their bodies may achieve limited positive changes. Others will experience a slowing down in the rate of debility. But for many, a reversal in their downward spiral is both to be anticipated and expected.

FORWARD LEAN

Problem:　Poor posture.

Exercises:　chest and hip flexor stretches, low back extensions, dumbbell rows, strengthening of the hip and back extensors, and posture tune-up: cervical glides (chapter 24), shoulders held slightly back, and a small arch in the low back maintained.

FORWARD FALL

Problem:　Poor posture and looking down.

Exercises:　Posture: see forward lean. An additional suggestion is to hold your head high and drop your chin. This permits you to look down without dropping your head and flexing the neck. When walking, concentrate on striking the heel with each step.

Shuffle Steps

Problem: Poor posture, weak or lazy hip flexors, and tight hip flexors. Problem may also be in the shoes—broken down or not laced up.

Exercises: An additional exercise is hip flexor strengthening (standing and sitting). Posture: see forward lean. See the exercise "Increasing Stride Length" at the end of this section. Try different shoes.

Short Steps

Problem: Fear of falling, possibly secondary to instability or insecurity.

Exercise: Maintain an upright posture and concentrate on the heel-strike phase of walking. You should already be planning on doing a lot of balance exercises. To help with your confidence, recruit an assistant who can walk beside you with a hand behind your upper arm. You may feel more secure and the light touch will not interfere with your balance.

Broad Base Gait

Problem: A balance problem exists. The broader base of support comes from the feet being farther apart. The push off from one foot creates both forward and opposite side momentum. There is very little stance time which eliminates the need to balance when walking. This is an inefficient and fatiguing walk.

Exercise: Balances especially on one leg.

EXCESSIVE TOE OUT

Problem: This is usually a sign of hip pathology. This can include results of surgery, arthritis, trauma, or prolonged bed confinement.

Exercise: Active hip internal rotations: Lie supine and roll both legs inwardly so your knee caps can look at each other. Work on balancing and on walking exercises while consciously keeping the toes pointing more straight ahead.

EXCESSIVE TOE IN (KNOCK KNEED)

Problem: Tightness in the hip internal rotators.

Exercise: Lie supine and roll both hips out at the same time. *Hold* for five seconds at the end of the roll. The tightness of the internal rotators acts as the resistance to strengthening the hip external rotators. When doing the balancing and walking exercises, consciously turn your foot more to the straight-ahead direction.

PAINFUL KNEES

Problem: It may or may not be a problem with the knee. If you had no knee pain until after you began a walking program, the problem may be in the foot.

Recommendation:

Shoe stores specializing in athletic footwear may be helpful in recommending an insert or possible a better shoe.

The other possibility is in the direction your feet are pointing when walking. Try a little toe in or toe out to see if this changes pain levels. A normal walk will not be possible in the presence of pain. A podiatrist is an excellent resource when it comes to managing foot problems.

Gluteus Medius Limp

Problem: Weakness in the muscle located on the side of the hip, causing a limp where the body dramatically tilts to the side of the stance leg.

This had been a common occurrence after total hip surgery, but the surgical techniques have changed and the frequency of this condition has dropped. Limps like this can trigger light headiness, can result in fatigue, and may contribute to the loss of balance and a fall. Are you hesitant to use a cane? The limp is much more obvious than the cane.

Exercise: Strengthen the muscle on the side of the hip in the direction of the tilt. Stand on the non affected leg and move the opposite leg to the side while keeping the leg from rolling outwardly. When standing on the left leg, the body tilts to the left, strengthen the left gluteus medius muscle. Also, put a cane in the right hand and advance it so that it remains touching the walking surface at all times when the left foot is touching.

Habitual Limp

Problem: Once a limp is established, the original cause may go away long before the limp.

Exercise: Maintain an upright posture and get into a position where you are able to see yourself walk. This feedback should encourage you to smooth out your walk. The "Increasing Stride Length" exercise may be helpful. But my favorite is retro-walking. This is walking backward where you have not established any bad habits. Find someone to assist you as a spotter. Don't look back when walking backward—you may lose your balance.

INCREASING STRIDE LENGTH

Exercise: Touch or hold on for balance until you are familiar and secure with this routine. Stand flat footed on the left and toe touching on the right. Step forward with the right landing on the heel. Shift all your weight onto the right flat foot, but keep the left toe in contact with the floor. Then shift your weight backward standing on the left leg momentarily as the right leg passes by.

The right toe makes contact behind you and the weight is shifted onto the right foot while the left heel remains touching the floor. Repeat this continuous forward and backward stepping in a short to normal stride length ten times with the right leg then do ten with the left twice a day.

WHAT WAS THAT CHAPTER ALL ABOUT?

Exercises are given for correcting walking problems.

Chapter 35

"WHAT IF I SHOULD FALL?"

I have an amazing ability to recover from potential falls. Yet, on two occasions, I felt helpless as I lay on the ground. By all rights, I could have fractured my lower leg in one fall and my hip in the other. Both were slips on black ice that I never saw coming. Perhaps if I weren't in such a hurry, they could have been prevented, or maybe not.

I am both convinced that virtually all falls can be prevented, and the chances are great that you and everyone you know have either fallen or will fall again.

Minimize those odds by improving your posture, strength, and balance. Also, personalize those commonsense principles contained in this publication. Assume they all apply to you! As a reminder, it may not be your *dog* that trips you up.

This chapter will address issues related to falling. Your familiarity with them may prevent a fall, minimize the severity of a fall, and prepare you to deal with the consequences of an actual fall.

SITTING DOWN AND GETTING OUT OF A CHAIR OR SOFA.

Deliberately and slowly descend to the sitting position, assisting with both your arms and legs, since sitting rapidly with minimal control can lead to a nasty fall.

In sitting down, turn around and back up until you feel the edge of the seat. If you have a weaker leg or one with limited knee or hip flexion (bending), put that leg forward as you reach back for the arm rest(s) with one or both hands.

To get up from a sitting position, slide forward on the seat. If possible, lean forward from the hips with your feet bent back and your heels a few inches behind your knees. Maintain your feet flat on the floor several inches apart.

As you push with your hands, your nose is above your toes. If one leg has limited flexion at the hip or knee, place it forward and push with the leg under you.

Push up with your palms on the arms of the chair so they take the weight. Your fingers are less likely to be able to take the strains. As you stand, straighten your knees and back at the same time.

Once upright, don't be in a hurry to walk away. You may want to take a step sideways to steady yourself. Arising too quickly may also result in a drop in blood pressure. Never begin walking if you sense that you are lightheaded.

Low Sofas or Easy Chairs

We all know that it is in our best interests to avoid those sofas that seem to swallow us up as we sink to the floor. Worse yet is to be trapped in the middle seat. At least with the outer seats you may have one over stuffed arm rest upon which to push. Don't let that hand slip, since directly beside that arm rest is an end table loaded with collectibles or chip dip.

The only way most Seniors have found to get up from the middle of a very low sofa is to scratch sideways to one of the arms and do a corkscrew and push ourselves up somehow. It's not a pretty sight. An option is to recruit someone to pull you up. If so, make sure you don't injure your helper or traumatize your own shoulders or arms.

The same issue applies to those chaise lounges popular at resort pools and summer gatherings. Worse yet, some of them have wheels making them even more hazardous when trying to get out.

When trapped into a chair without arms, one technique is to grab the seat between your legs and push up with arms and legs as you lean forward. If possible, recruit a spotter to assist you if you should need it.

The best advice is to avoid the whole thing. As you enter the room, head directly for the higher chair with arms. If you don't see it, ask for one. Use arm chairs at the pool or picnic.

PRACTICING HOW TO FALL ON A LEVEL SURFACE

Falls often happen too fast for us to react until they're over. The bright side is that there wasn't time to get tense. A stiff body breaks while a limp body bends.

On the other hand, if you feel yourself falling, try to relax, lower your center of gravity by bending your knees, and attempt to break your fall by grabbing on to something stable.

You can practice every night by falling into bed, first in a sitting position and then forward as well as onto your sides. Perfecting the art of falling includes both knowing how to land as well as how to relax in the process.

I have taught individuals to fall, and we practiced on well padded floor mats.

FALLING DOWN A STAIRS

I have never instructed anyone, or know anyone who has, how to fall on stairs safely. My advice to everyone, regardless of age and physical condition, is to use the handrails every time.

AVOIDING THE WORST INJURIES

Focusing on remaining upright is much more pleasant than on deciding which body part we would prefer to injure should we fall, but someday it may come to this.

Few would disagree that closed head trauma ranks at the top of falling's worst-injury list. We must protect our heads at all costs even if it results in a skinned elbow or fractured wrist.

The fall least likely to cause injury is backward onto your buttocks. If that's the direction you are heading, tuck the chin to avoid striking the back of your head.

If you are falling forward, keep your chin up and break the fall with your arms and hands.

Fractured hips rank second on the worst-injury list. These usually result from landing sideways directly on the hip. Unfortunately, you have few options for breaking a fall to the side.

IF YOU FALL

After a fall, don't be in a hurry to get up. Forget the embarrassment of the moment, lie still, and take inventory.

Are you experiencing pain, and is there any obvious deformity? Does movement of the injured body part increases the pain? If so, don't attempt to get up, and don't eat and drink until you are medically checked out. This is in the event you need surgery.

If you suspect a serious injury, don't let anyone move you and wait for a paramedic. If no one is around and you have a cell phone, call 911, a friend, or a family member.

GETTING UP AFTER A FALL

Falling down just happens, but you need a plan to get up. Once you have determined that you are not seriously injured, it's time to get up.

First of all, free up both hands and clear the area of objects you may have been carrying so you don't trip over them.

Crawl to a chair or other stable object that you can use to steady yourself. Roll onto your strong side or one that allows you to bend your stronger knee.

The following directions are for those who roll onto their left side. Put your right hand flat in front of you at belt level and push so your shoulders are off the floor and your weight is on your left hip.

Roll forward onto your knees using your hands for support. With your hands on the secure object, lift a knee so your leg is bent and foot flat on the floor. Now, pull yourself up.

This technique is not recommended for those Seniors who have had a hip replacement. Better to wait for assistance even if you are not seriously injured.

In Case of Emergency

When a TV show can give a contestant three life lines, we Seniors owe it to ourselves to have at least one. For use in emergencies, cell phones are user friendly and can be carried everywhere.

One suggestion is to put ICE (in case of emergency) in the name section. Speed dial #2 can be programmed to the person you would want contacted in an emergency. Or you can call 911.

The wireless cell phone companies and local governments are beginning to set up Global Positioning Satellite system tied into 911 calls. It's on all the new cell phones.

If the local government has enhanced 911 capabilities, when we dial 911, even if we say nothing, the authorities can zero in on our location within 150 meters, which is about 167 yards. To find out if your local public safety answering system has this capability, check the National Emergency Number Association at www.nena.org.

Some may wish to consider buying into a personal emergency response system. These medical alarms are small devices worn around the neck or wrist. You need only press a button to get help.

What Was That Chapter All About?

Many childhood injuries occur because of inability to anticipate danger. As Seniors, we seem to recognize the danger but sometimes choose to ignore it. This includes unwise seating selections, walking before fully standing, thinking that your dizziness will pass, and a personal belief that cell phones are exclusively for the younger generation.

Nobody is immune to falling, but honing your anticipation skills may prevent an avoidable mishap. On the other hand, in the event that one day you do fall, you will want to be prepared to assist yourself or to direct others on your behalf.

Chapter 36

ALTERNATIVE ACTIVITIES

Not everyone can or will want to incorporate a walking routine into their rehabilitation program. The following activities may appeal to some. Keep in mind that it is far better to be *doing* something than to be *thinking* about doing everything.

There are programs that incorporate meditation and others are recreational in nature. Neither should be confused with aerobic activities that are done at least three times a week which increase respiration, heart rate, etc.

BODY, MIND, AND SPIRIT

Yoga. Is a form of physical and mental meditation that seeks an awareness of a deeper understanding of self. Yoga utilizes mostly mats, is performed in positions free from the risk of falling, and facilitates efficient breathing patterns. Yoga can also be adapted to enhance on balance.

Pilates. Incorporates a series of low impact flexibility and muscular and endurance exercises utilizing machines, bars, belts, and/or balls. Pilates gradually rebuilds confidence, core muscles, and postural awareness.

Tai Chi. Performed in a calm environment incorporating slow and controlled choreographed movements. Tai Chi has been shown to improve single-leg standing, to slow down walking speed, and thus reduce the risk of falling. Tai Chi programs can be specifically geared for Seniors.

RECREATIONAL ACTIVITIES

Bicycling. Many of us learned on a tricycle, and now they're marketing the adult version to Seniors. When balance is an issue, the stability of the third wheel is welcomed. There is minimal impacting forces on the weight bearing joints, but those with hip or knee pathology may find bikes as being either therapeutic or "killers." Try one out before buying it.

Swimming. Do your knees hurt too much to walk or bike? Try swimming. The "Y" may have a pool and many schools provide times for open swims. These pools may also be warm to accommodate arthritic individuals. Retirement communities may market their pools as an incentive for living there.

Ask about water aerobics. They provide an excellent opportunity to exercise in an environment where falling does not pose a risk. Lap swimming is a good conditioning exercise if you have that talent and can find a lap lane or pool.

Jogging. Even at 5 mph, jogging is rated as a moderately high-calorie-burning activity. That's why you don't see many happy joggers. Unless you have been an accomplished runner or jogger in the recent past, don't even think about it.

Dancing. "Mayo Clinic researchers report that dancing can help reduce stress, increase energy, improve strength and increase muscle tone and coordination." The *National Heart, Lung and Blood Institute* credits dancing with lowering the risk of coronary heart disease, decreasing blood pressure, and managing weight.

A study published by the *New England Journal of Medicine* noted that dancing can lower the risk of Alzheimer's disease and other dementia-type conditions in other adults. See "MHS Connections," Fall 2007.

Are you concerned about your balance but are interested in dancing? Hold on to your partner.

Fishing. This can be an active or a passive activity. The challenge of fly fishing or the calm of dangling a line are both therapeutic to those who engage in them. However, standing on a boat deck, whether fishing or not, can be a real balancing experience.

Sitting. You probably shouldn't know about this, but just sitting around burns some calories. Want to burn more? Sit in a rocking chair.

Horseback Riding. This activity has been successfully incorporated into the developmental programs for physically challenged children. Given the proper environment, Seniors could consider sitting in the saddle of a moving horse also to be therapeutic. The unexpected movements induce the core muscles to continuously contract as balance checks. But beware; falling off can be fatal.

Golf. Providing you walk the course, golf can provide moderate exercise, even if it drives you crazy. A golf swing and the walking challenge both the extremity and core muscles. It is also a good idea to work on your flexibility before swinging a club.

Bowling. Check with your local bowling centers regarding Senior leagues. The minimum age is usually fifty-five and many are held during the day. The rates are usually less, and if you're lucky, maybe there will be free coffee.

Bowling combines socialization and competition, plus, physiologically, it enhances balance coordination, mobility, and strength. Sounds like a sales pitch? Consider the following from *Ten Pin Talk* (January 1, 2007):

1. Bowlers use 134 muscles during the basic four step approach.
2. An average bowler swings 864 pounds full circle in a three-game series.
3. Three games of bowling equals walking one mile.
4. The average adult bowler burns 240 calories per hour.

Gardening. Many Seniors find gardening as a good recreational activity, but it is especially stressful for the unsteady. Leaning over and reaching down for prolonged periods of time are typical postures assumed by many gardeners.

To reduce the associated stresses, consider the following suggestions. Use kneeling pads, stools, long handled tools, patio or flower boxes, elevated garden beds, and/or hanging baskets.

HOUSEHOLD CHORES

These may not be considered recreational, but they do burn calories and do involve moderate exercise.

Mowing the lawn. Walking behind a self-propelled mower provides a moderate amount of exercise, plus it allows you to hold on to a handle for balance assistance as you maneuver over soft and possible irregular surfaces.

Doing housework. Housekeeping is a purposeful activity that burns calories and incorporates flexibility, strength, and balance skills. There may not be difficult to make it more enjoyable, but the challenge is to enhance the safety factor for unsteady Seniors.

One suggestion is to pace yourself. Do no more than fifteen to twenty minutes at one time or during one day. Space your housekeeping activity to last all week.

Another helpful hint is to hold on to something to assist your balance. If it is running a vacuum cleaner, don't trip over the cord. If you want a challenge, hold on to the vacuum with the other hand.

Avoid looking up. In the kitchen move items you regularly access to lower shelves. If you must use a ladder, go no higher than two steps and use a step ladder with an attached hand grip.

Avoid looking down with your neck. Refer to the posture chapter 24 on how to look down with your head and eyes.

Do these housework activities when you have the most amount of light.

Hire out the more strenuous and difficult jobs.

Removing snow. It is better to use a snow blower than a shovel unless the snow is so wet that it clogs. In that case, pay someone to do it.

COMPUTERIZED BALANCE TRAINING WITH WII DEVICES

These are interactive video activities similar to those used to simulate playing golf or bowling. The participant stands on a force plate and follows the instructions on a monitor. The device permits you to progress at a safe and controlled pace, and they also give you immediate feedback by generating scores for each session.

For those who are interested, I suggest you contact physical therapy clinics/departments and ask them if they are using a Wii balance and assessment device. Remember, it's best to try it before you buy it.

LITTLE ADD-ONS

Every day, there are activities that Seniors can do to increase their physical expenditures without significantly altering their lifestyle. These are referred to as the little add-ons.

Betsy Stephens addressed several of these in an article she wrote in the March-April 2003 issue of the *AARP Magazine*. I added some others. Consider each one as a suggestion and only adopt those that may work for you.

Taking stairs instead of elevators is a perennial favorite that's loaded with disclaimers. I'm not fond of any exercise that uses stairs. Things to consider are the condition of your hips, knees, and ankles, your general physical fitness and the added stress to your heart.

Also, do these stairs have secure railings, and are they well lit and maintained? Stairways in public buildings are not always easily found, and how many times do you only go up or down one level?

Parking away from the front door of an establishment will let you walk a little farther and perhaps spare your doors from some dings. Use common sense when it comes to personal safety. Consider this activity when you have a companion and/or when other people are around. Do not do this at night or when the parking lots are in disrepair.

You may consider getting off the bus one stop earlier.

Stand at a counter top as you read the newspaper. Today, you make it through section A and maybe, in six months, the whole paper.

When shopping in the mall, get what you came for and then take a little extra walk afterward. If you are in a grocery store, go midmorning when it is less busy and walk around pushing your cart before checking out.

At home, stand during the TV commercials and practice shifting your weight from leg to leg. Also, walk around your uncluttered home during your casual phone conversations. You may also set an alarm on your wristwatch or cell phone to remind you that each hour your kitchen or main floor needs to be patrolled.

Brushing your teeth is a once-or-more-a-day event that you could consider for a little add-on. One well-meaning youngster suggested standing on one foot as you brush, but I don't think much of that.

Bending forward while brushing can stress the back. Try leaning forward onto one hand or forearm while brushing with the other. Keep one leg under you with the other slightly to the rear. If both legs are equally strong, alternate supporting legs.

Betsy has a perverse sense of humor when she suggested that for one week we hide the TV remote. Perhaps this would get us Seniors out of our easy chairs and into some other kind of activity.

Little add-ons may become part of your daily routine. However, if you are unable to relate to any of these, maybe there are others better suited for you. Your imagination is the limit tempered by commonsense.

WHAT WAS THAT CHAPTER ALL ABOUT?

Alternative activities can be effective complementary additions to rehabilitation programs. Continue with the exercises targeting specific deficiencies, but add a little recreation. Working on your balance program may improve your "game," but participating in an alternative activity can promote your balance skills. This is called cross training and often is worth a try.

Chapter 37

DESIGNING YOUR EXERCISE PROGRAM

By this time, you should have a good idea of your specific needs, and I never cease to be amazed at what people can accomplish on their own.

But if you feel overwhelmed by the task lying ahead, perhaps you should begin by getting professional insight, like from a physical therapist.

PLANNING A MANAGEABLE ROUTINE

On the other hand, if you are ready to plan your own program, start with a manageable routine both with respect to the physical demands on your body and with consideration of any time constraints.

Be familiar with the recommended number of holds, reps, and sets put forth in each of the exercise chapters. But establishing a program specific to your needs may require the tweaking of these guidelines.

As a word of caution, being overly aggressive initially may be counterproductive. A faithful commitment to a few exercises is far better than good intentions to do many and haphazardly following through.

USE YOUR TEST RESULTS AS A GUIDE

Tests, unlike exercises, are conducted on an infrequent basis, like every month or two. Therefore, maintain these records separately from your exercise logs and diaries. Also include in this file any tests and test results performed by your physician or health-care professionals.

As a reminder, every effort must be made to minimize testing variables. This includes reassessing your posture prior to retesting your flexibility, strength, and balance. Guidelines for testing consistencies were covered in the Balance-Challenged chapter.

As you consider which exercises to include in your program, should you skip all that posture, breathing, stretching, and strengthening, and just concentrate on those maneuvers used to test balance?

That's like doing well on your final exam because you had it in advance to study. You may score well on your Stork and Walk-in-Line tests but your functional balance remains impaired.

Tweaking does not mean taking shortcuts. None of us has achieved perfection even in one area, but we all know that some things need more work than others.

Organizing Your Exercise Program

Begin by making a list of exercises you feel belong in your program. Then categorize them according to posture/breathing, stretching, strengthening, balance, and conditioning.

Posture and breathing tune-up. Each session will begin with posture tune-up and breathing exercises. Do as many as you feel are necessary to prepare you for the exercises to follow—stretching, strengthening, and ending with balancing techniques. These represent the foundational components of your rehabilitation program.

Conditioning. The ultimate goal of this program is the resumption of functional activities such as walking. One step farther is to use activities such as walking for conditioning. However, it is not necessary to incorporate them with the foundational exercises until it is safe to do so.

Logical ordering. It will be necessary to organize each list into a logical order, but more on that later. The next section will provide you with additional exercising insights.

An Exercise Overview

Bed stretches when you wake up. Don't be in a hurry to get up each morning. If the knee-to-chest stretches are therapeutic for you, lie on one side and/or the other and rest with one or both knees raised toward your chest. On the other hand, if back extensions feel good, lie on your stomach for a while. These are rest positions, so do them as long as they feel good.

The chapter "Guidelines for Stretching," detailed many stretches that can be performed in bed. There is no harm in doing some of these now, or you can wait and do the ones that are on tap for the exercises that day. Daily stretching can be therapeutic, and I wouldn't want you to miss an opportunity.

Stretching benefits. Morning stiffness is a predictable condition especially in pathological joints (those affected by disease or injury). But regardless of the reason, stretching and range of motion exercise done before breakfast can act as a wake-up call to our bodies.

Stretching to regain joint mobility is a formidable challenge, especially at the Senior level. The benefits of stretching prior to strengthening specific muscles have not been validated by studies. Gentle stretching after strengthening has been shown to reduce post exercise tightness and soreness.

Gradual warm-up and cool-down phases to a conditioning activity seem to be more effective than stretching.

In short, the effectiveness of stretching is determined by each individual. Record responses in your exercise diary, and don't be afraid to try different routines to find what is best for you.

Strengthening exercises. To get the most out of the strengthening program, adhere to the guidelines for strengthening set forth in chapter 31.

Prepare a list of all the strengthening exercises you plan on doing and divide them into two groups, each to be done on alternate days. For example, on Monday, Wednesday, and Friday, concentrate on the quads, hamstrings, lower legs (ankles), and feet. On Tuesday, Thursday, and Saturday, strengthen the core muscles (back, abdominals, and hips) plus any arm exercises.

When establishing the order in which to do the exercises, consider the positions you will be in. Do all those you can while standing, then to sitting, and lastly lying down.

Using this approach will put you in the standing position when most rested and lying down when most fatigued. It also varies the specific muscles being worked on which will help reduce muscular fatigue. One last benefit is that it also uses your exercise time more efficiently.

To organize the program, take one piece of paper and list the "standing" group of exercises then the "sitting" group and then the "lying down" group in the vertical column.

The horizontal column is for the dates. Depending upon how many exercises you have, you could use one sheet for *M, W, F* and another for *Tu, Th, Sa*. This may provide you with enough space at the bottom for comments.

If you adhere to the same exercise protocol each day, say three sets of ten reps, then all you need in the corresponding boxes is the resistance. Check marks are okay if no changes were made from the previous day's workout.

Balancing exercises. Balancing is an art form, not a repetitive activity. One done well is far better than many performed poorly.

Each balance exercise targets a different compensatory mechanism. Since individuals are unique, so are their needs. The time of day, which balances are incorporated into the program, and how many of each are done are all variables to be determined by each of you.

To organize the process, take one piece of paper and list all the balance exercises in the vertical column, in no particular order. Once you are more familiar with them, you could rearrange them according to the time of day or in conjunction with another activity, i.e. doing the dishes, brushing teeth, after exercising, while watching the evening news, etc.

On the horizontal, across the top of the page, put in the days of the month. Each time you complete a balance exercise, check it off in the corresponding box. You may even get several checks in one box. Practice regularity is important, and, at the end of the day, all boxes will have at least one check mark.

Conditioning exercise. Conditioning exercises are structured activities that can be pursued seven days a week. A partial list includes walking on the treadmill, riding the stationary bike, using the elliptical trainer as well as bike riding and walking outside the home.

You could be working on more than one of these conditioning exercises, but no more than one a day is recommended. For example, walk outside on the good days and on the treadmill on bad weather days. Or you can alternate days between riding and walking.

Documentation, once again, is important. List the activity in the vertical column and the dates horizontally. Daily achievements go in the corresponding boxes.

Being unsteady by no means exempts you from conditioning. Begin with an activity that you feel comfortably safe in doing. As your strength, endurance, and balance improve, you may consider changing activities.

It is also conceivable that many of you will achieve super Senior status and progress to the level of an intense exercise, like power walking or singles tennis. If you should, limit your participation to three times a week.

WRITING OUT YOUR PROGRAM

In the physical therapy profession, as with all medical disciplines, if a procedure was done and not documented, in the eyes of auditors—*It wasn't done! It didn't happen!*

Accurate records are necessary to assure quality care. What a client accomplishes on one day dictates the course of action on the next visit.

Health clubs encourage their customers to complete a workout record for each session. Personal trainers also maintain detailed files on everyone they work with.

Adopt the same mentality when it comes to your own exercise routine. By doing so, you can maintain a consistent exercise sequence; you can build on previous accomplishments; you can accurately reproduce self-testing techniques, and you can see progress over the course of many sessions.

I can't remember the last time I forgot anything. That's a joke! Try exercising without keeping written records, and you will soon find out how little you retain from day to day. What began as a well intentioned workout will end in an exercise of frustration.

The rewards of detailed documentation will pay dividends beyond expectation. They will also be a record of additions and/or deletions as you fine tune or progress.

Exercise flow sheets. All those sheets you filled out with vertical and horizontal columns are called flow sheets. They keep you organized by indicating which exercise comes next, the level of intensity, and keep you from forgetting any exercise.

An exercise diary. Comment on any aspect of a specific exercise session and use these insights to help with subsequent workouts. Possible entries are: "too aggressive on hamstring stretches," "increase resistance on the leg lifts," "the red and white shoes are best for walking," and "I didn't lose my balance once today."

Date each entry since the exercise diary may be kept separate from the exercise sheets. The more you put into it, the greater benefit you will get out of it.

WHAT WAS THAT CHAPTER ALL ABOUT?

Exercise is one of those activities that you need to participate in to appreciate its benefits. Exercising with a friend may enhance your compliance and enjoyment levels, but adhere to your workout regime, not theirs.

Maintain your records with a compulsive mind-set. Details are important to assess progress as well as to dictate when to change.

Recreational activities done on an irregular basis should not replace exercises on your workout sheet.

Chapter 38

SOME FINAL THOUGHTS

During my undergraduate studies in Physical Education, a professor intimidated us with this remark, "If you think that you are a good teacher, teach yourself to play a sport with the opposite hand."

I never felt guilty about not taking him up on his challenge, but I remain humbled by the enormity of doing that kind of project.

Imagine learning all those new motor skills. But that is what rehabilitation is all about.

For some, it is relearning how to roll over, sit, and stand, and for others, it is how to remain standing once there.

Initially, the entire process may seem overwhelming, but focus on the fact that the restoration of balance in Seniors is an attainable goal.

I came across this quote from Bruce Barton that appeared in the *Reader's Digest* many years ago: "Nothing splendid has even been achieved except by those who dared believe that something inside them was superior to circumstance." So "Life isn't about waiting for the storm to pass. It's about learning to dance in the rain."

PART THREE

A REFERENCE FILE OF
USEFUL INFORMATION

These are the kind of things that are useful to know about; however, at our age or at any other age, we can't be expected to always keep them straight in our heads.

Chapter 39

Supports: Canes, Walkers, Braces

Some Seniors only feel safe if they use a cane all of the time. Others use a cane once in a while. Put a check for Charlie in that second box. Each of us should listen to our knees and bodies and let them tell us when it's a good idea to reach for a balance check or even a little extra support in emergencies.

What the Supports Can Do

One purpose of the various supports such as canes is that they help us unsteady types walk more like other people, what the experts call a normal gait pattern. The light touch gives us a sense of our position in space.

Canes

Canes are used for balance. This "third leg" acts to widen our support base beyond our two feet, and by touching, they help steady us.

Using a cane reduces the amount of weight you put on a painful foot or weak leg by about 25 percent. Walkers with their wider base of support, and crutches are more effective in helping reduce more weight bearing, with the arms taking more of the weight.

Shopping for a Cane

Canes can be found in grocery stores, pharmacies, medical supply houses, online, at flea markets, and estate sales to name a few. There is a vast variety of styles out there.

Choosing a standard-type cane. With shoes on and hands hanging loosely at your side, you should see the top of the rubber-tipped cane at the crease where your hand and wrist join. The cane should be placed three inches from your foot and you should, of course, wear the shoes you normally do.

Wood or aluminum? The advantage of aluminum over wooden canes is they are lighter, and they usually can be adjusted for height. They also offer a wider selection of handle types. With wood or fiberglass canes, you take the length they have or have to saw them to the proper length.

Cane Handles. Handles are offset, flat, or curved. The offset provide more stability. Choose what feels best. Those Seniors with arthritis may find a curved crook handle painful.

These old fashioned curved ones have a candy-cane-type handle. A standard style widely popular is shaped like an upside-down *L*. It's called a Fritz Handle—don't ask; we don't know. It provides a longer support surface and greater hand comfort. A *T* shape distributes the weight on the shaft more efficiently.

Swan necked or offset types are designed to place the hand directly over the shaft, which permits the user to push down harder. And there are ergonomic handles that take less strength to grip since they are shaped to fit the contours of one's hand. Others are designed for those with smaller hands. And some have grips that can be adjusted to different angles.

Added features on standard canes. Many canes have handle straps that help keep us from dropping them. Some have handles that spread apart and give you a place to sit on when tired.

Rubber tips on our canes get worn down faster than you may think and can be easily replaced.

Retractable tips to navigate on ice are available. They can be attached to canes and walkers in winter.

And there are tips that allow you to place the cane in a stand-up position. Some allow you to pick up a fallen cane by stepping on a side of the tip.

And then there are those splendid, special added features. Most practical are those with a special cushioning grip of felt or foam to the handle, making it easier to hold.

One practical innovation is a cane that stores an extra grip that you can insert into the shaft to provide leverage if you need help getting up from a kneeling position.

Still, as we write, you can even buy a "walking stick" with a handle that has a carved Sherlock Holmes bust. It just costs just eighty-five dollars. Or you can just spend your eighty-five dollars on something foolish.

You can buy fancy canes in different colors and with tiger or other fabric handles and even with jewels embedded. A woman friend has one that looks like it's made out of glass, with her name on it, and every five inches or so one of those happy faces.

Some of the snazzier canes will hold your car keys. You can also now get a cane with a built-in alarm button, a red safety signal, a tag that lists your medical needs, a light that shines ahead for six feet, and, we kid you not, a built-in massager for your back. This "multiwalking stick" will support up to eight hundred pounds and can be taken apart for packing.

A special bed cane can be strapped on to the bed frame and is available for those who have trouble getting out of bed because of recent surgery or general weakness.

Using a Standard Cane

As we walk, our elbow should be bent slightly—fifteen to thirty degrees. We can get that if we divide a ninety-degree right angle into thirds or sixths. The arm opposite the cane swings forward as we step out.

If we are using a cane to take a little weight off a weak leg, we should hold the cane on the opposite side of the weak limb. The cane always moves at the same time as the weak leg.

You should avoid putting the cane too far ahead.

Going up a stairs, always keep the cane with the weak leg. This means going up as well as down the stairs. When going up stairs, leading with the strong leg and following with the weak leg and the cane is best. However, leading with the weak limb and the cane is also acceptable but may seem contradictory to the reader. The cane should remain with the weak limb just for extra support if needed.

Cane tips. Check tips to see if they are worn. Once, Charlie put a metal chair tip on the end of his cane. They are cheaper but don't have the quality or durability of a cane tip. They also slip more easily on wet and tile surfaces. The plastic chair tip was white rather than the harder nonskid black or gray of regular cane tips.

Drying the cane tip, perhaps on a rug, when coming in from the rain is a good idea. If not, be especially wary on linoleum, tile, or on those marble-type floors often found in banks and public buildings.

You might also want to check when coming in from the snow since snow caught up in the grooves of the cane tip can turn to ice when it hits a warm surface.

Using Two Standard Canes

This technique is especially useful after a leg operation, for winter walking, and also for fast walking. See Don's section on Nordic canes.

Three- or Four-Legged (Quad) Canes

Quad canes require a person to walk very slowly to keep all four points in contact with the floor at one time. If you are able to walk faster safely, you would be better off switching to a standard cane. Trying to walk fast with a quad cane may lead to balance and support problems.

Aluminum canes with a tripod or quad base provide greater stability, and they can stand up alone, freeing your hands. Going up steps, however, is more difficult than with a standard cane.

The flat edge of a quad cane base should be closest to your body.

Fold Up Canes and Canes That Unscrew into Sections

These are helpful when traveling since they fit inside luggage and can be an extra cane in case you mislay one. However they can't take as much weight in an emergency as standard canes and aren't recommended for regular use.

The canes that come apart sometimes get loose and may need a piece of paper around the screws to keep them tight.

Sit-Down Canes

You can get canes without a spear end. Charlie's brother-in-law, the orthopod, made him buy one of these after a knee operation. They may be made out of metal and make quite a weapon. Charlie still remembers a Sunday at a deserted train station in London when a man with what looked like a hangover came along muttering unpleasant things about Americans, but that's another story.

Walkers

When should you use a walker? You'll know. It's when you have generalized weakness.

They have some disadvantages: They are hard to navigate in tight places, and those with wheels can't be used on stairs. Your walk and posture may change, by using shorter steps and bending over. Not all walkers fold up or can be adjusted for the proper height.

The standard walker without wheels has four solid legs with rubber tips and gives a larger base of support than a cane. It needs to be lifted completely off the ground at each step.

Two wheeled walkers make walking easier but are less stable but still provide a larger base of support than a cane. Up to 50 percent of your weight may be put on the front wheels. The larger the wheels, the smoother they run. The back legs on some have tennis balls or ski tips which allow them to slide along. They cannot be used on stairs.

Four wheeled walkers are mainly used for balance since they're not intended to take weight. There's always the danger that they may flip. They cannot be used on stairs.

Some walkers have a seat, a basket, and a tail light—just kidding about the light. There are also fancy and expensive walkers with padded seats, backrests, and brakes.

CRUTCHES

Their main function is to avoid putting weight on a compromised lower extremity.

The type we normally think of extends to the armpit and is called the axillary crutch. They can be wooden or aluminum. The axillary pad should come within the width of three fingers below the armpit.

The forearm or Canadian crutches have forearm cuffs and hand grips. The cuff should reach to one and a half inches below the elbow. The handgrip should be level with the crease in your palm.

Canadian crutches are aluminum, support less weight than standard crutches but allow you to use both hands without putting the crutches down. Gaining proficiency with them may take longer.

Regardless of the style of crutch, upper body strength and unimpaired balance skills are necessary. If you don't qualify, opt instead for a walker.

MEDICARE COVERAGE

The cost of canes, crutches, and walkers may be covered when a doctor prescribes them. Check your insurance benefits to be sure.

ANKLE OR KNEE BRACES (ORTHOTICS)

Braces are used to provide external support to a body part that is no longer capable of performing its intended function. This may be from weakness, instability, or paralysis. If the purpose is to compensate for weakness, you are then obliged to adhere to a strengthening program for the compromised muscles. If not, the weaker get weaker.

Braces vary by their intended use. They can be slipped on, Velcro secured, or fancy ones with metal side supports and hinges. Regardless, these are prescribed items by medical experts.

ELASTIC WRAPS

Wraps provide psychological support, uneven pressure, and don't stay in place. After a while, when you look down, you may find them twisted around your ankles. It's a mystery how those World War I doughboys kept those puttees up to pass inspection.

Some wraps come with Velcro closures while others have special little clasps that tend to fall off. I put tape over the clasps to prevent them from getting lost.

Neoprene elastic sleeves. These are commonly used to reduce swelling through compression, to improve your sense of position, and to provide warmth. However, many Seniors are allergic to neoprene.

Patellar stabilization braces. These are designed to stabilize knee caps, but their effectiveness is not universal. Straps anchor the brace, and some allow the wearer to replace the straps that wear out. Others have Velcro straps. Some provide a static pressure, while others, called dynamic braces, vary the pressure on the knee cap. The hinges on braces at the knee joint should be covered to protect from rubbing.

Patellar instability is a condition that can lead both to falling and inactivity. These braces can be purchased in medical supply stores and some pharmacies.

Unloading braces. These braces are designed to correct poor body alignment and reduce pain. They are helpful for Seniors with osteoarthritis and can be ordered after your doctor takes precise measurements. Insurance may cover the cost when a physician prescribes them.

Functional braces. These are designed to provide stability to those with arthritis and ligament problems. Custom-made supports will fit better and are less likely to slip. Others can be purchased at pharmacies. Insurance may cover them if ordered by a physician.

AKROD v2 Robotic Knee Brace. This brace uses sensors and what the manufacturers call smart fluid to vary the resistance on the joints during walking. The brace was developed at Northeastern University and was going through human trials several years ago.

The BioniCare BIOC1000 Stimulator. This device is a brace designed to strengthen the knee joint while sleeping. It consists of a battery-powered signal generator, two electrode pads (One covers the knee; the other rests on the thigh.), and a Velcro wrap that holds the pads in place.

Those who have tried them have reported improvements in range of motion, reduced pain, and stiffness. Maximum relief may take up to five months. They are also used after knee replacements and are available for purchase.

Programmable rehabilitative braces. Dr. Constantinos Mavroidis, an associate professor of Mechanical and Industrial Engineering at Northeastern University in Boston, and his students have added a small gadget to braces. When a computer electrically charges the brace, it creates resistance, just like a weight exercise machine. The resistance can be programmed at different levels for different activities from walking to stair climbing.

It is not yet available for purchase (an estimated five-year release date), but, in case you are interested, it will probably sell at two thousand dollars. The device, when on the market, will be run on batteries. The big advantage seems to be that you get continuous resistance exercise all day long.

SHOE INSERTS

Up until now, we have said little about a very helpful professional consultant—the podiatrist. There are numerous bodily ailments originating from insufficiently supported feet, and they are the experts.

One type of support is an Orthotic, which are custom-made shoe inserts and arch supports fitted to your individual needs. These are expensive but very durable and can be removed and replaced in other shoe ware. Some insurance plans will pay for one set per lifetime.

Of course, you also can find those less expensive over-the-counter inserts. They tend to be thicker on the inside edge, which makes them more suitable for those who are slightly knock-kneed and not as helpful for those who are slightly bowlegged.

Gait Analysis

A friend of Charlie described her experience at a gait analysis center. They visually analyzed her walking patterns, measured muscle activity patterns, joint motion, and oxygen consumption, filmed her, put her data into a computer, and also took X-rays of her bone formation. The result was a specially designed shoe insert, which she says helped. The cost was around five hundred dollars.

A Stabilizer for Winter Weather

The Yaktrax walkers slip over your shoe just like those old-fashioned rubbers. It is a plastic net crisscrossed with high-strength steel. A pair costs around twenty dollars. Studies indicate that Seniors with balance problems benefit from the added traction.

Choosing Shoes

Exercise shoes should be replaced at least once a year if used regularly especially for outside walking. Check for wear pattern on the bottom of the shoes.

Different foot problems require different types of shoes. Your arch may have collapsed and rolls inward when you walk; this is called over pronation. Or it may roll to the outside of your foot, which is called supination. Each requires a different kind of support. Consult a specialist prior to purchasing a shoe.

Different exercise activities also require different shoes. Running and walking shoes are different for example.

Many experts recommend those white athletic shoes (sneakers) for Seniors for everyday wear. You can clean them with Windex. A study of 1371 people aged sixty-five and older found those wearing athletic shoes were 30 percent less likely to fall. So reports *Arthritis Today* in their April 2006 issue.

Some leisure-type shoes have Velcro straps or buckles that do away with laces. It also helps to have tops that stretch somewhat so they can mold around the feet.

Unsteady Seniors should buy shoes that are light. Choose flat heeled shoes, even high-topped models with nonskid thin soles. Thick heavy soles encourage falls. Avoid leather soles; they slip. The sole should be flexible at the ball of the foot rather in the middle.

Rubber cushions are recommended. The arch support should fill up the middle of the arch. The shoe should fit snugly at the heels to prevent rubbing up and down. Check for seams inside that may rub.

Do not to trust size figures on the shoe, but we perhaps knew that already. Rather, we should see how the shoe feels. It should have a wide toe box, with a half inch from toe to shoe, so we can wiggle our toes. The shoes should also have a no-slip back.

In an article in *Diabetes Forecast* on August 2006, Shauna Roberts suggested we outline our bare feet on a piece of thin paper and place any shoe we may be thinking of buying on it. Or we can measure both feet and buy for the larger.

Stand up when trying on shoes since feet expand when you stand. Buy shoes late in the day; the foot expands as the day goes on.

THE MASAI BAREFOOT TECHIT

This is a peculiar sneaker, very popular in Europe, and is turning up here as well. A Swiss engineer named Karl Muller, a former semiprofessional footballer, invented it after watching the relaxed, long, striding Masai of East Africa as they covered uneven ground. At least that's what he claims.

From the top, the MBT looks like a regular sneaker, but the sole is two inches thick and tapers sharply from the middle to the toe. As you walk, you will roll forward.

Muller claims that normal flat soled-shoes lead to lazy walking and poor posture. The MBT encourages rock and roll to the toe and is supposed to relieve joint pain by strengthening our thigh muscles. And those who have tried them found the MBT also reduces weight; in other words, you have to work harder when you wear them.

It doesn't sound like this invention is designed for unsteady Seniors, and besides it costs $250. Still, it's good to be up on the latest, just in case one of your grand offspring tries to hit you up for "just a pair of MBT sneakers for Christmas."

The Step Stretch. This is a stationary rocker that we can place one foot on and rock back and forth to strengthen the same muscles that the MBT does. It sells for around forty dollars.

CHOOSING SOCKS

Again, the experts have a recommendation for Seniors' high-tech athletic socks made of synthetic acrylic materials. They absorb sweat, cushion well, and protect feet from friction.

CHOOSING AN EASY CHAIR

The depth of the seat is a critical factor; too shallow causes excessive posterior thigh pressure, and too deep promotes a slouching posture. Mutt and Jeff couples may need him and her chairs. We should try a chair for at least twenty minutes to make sure it's what we want.

No chair fits everyone. We have differences. We all want to avoid chairs that are too low and too hard for us to get out of or chairs too high that will not allow our feet to touch the floor. We also should avoid chairs so narrow that we can't move around and relieve stiffness.

We need one with a firm cushion but with a little give. We don't want one that causes us to sink down with our rear end below our knees and makes it difficult for us to get up or so firm as to make us stiff and uncomfortable.

It should be just deep enough so it will support our upper legs but no more. The chair should allow two to three inches between our calves and its front. The back should support our entire back including shoulders and neck. The arm rests should be high enough so we can rest our whole lower arm when seated. Some chairs are adjustable. If you become heir to a chair that is all wrong for you, chuck it. It can cause discomfort and real problems.

Lift chairs are available and Medicare Part B will pay some of the costs if a doctor orders one for you.

WHAT WAS THAT CHAPTER ALL ABOUT?

We have listed the choices available and what the experts recommend in canes, walkers, crutches, braces, shoes, shoe inserts, socks, and easy chairs.

Chapter 40

COMMON INJURIES: TREATMENT AND MEDICATIONS

Seniors, more than any other population group except perhaps kids, are involved in medical situations, from the serious to the just aggravating. We try to cover the waterfront of sports injuries.

IF YOU SUSPECT THAT A FALL MAY BE SERIOUS

Severe pain may be the tip off. Call 911 for a paramedic immediately.

Don't move but have someone keep you warm with blankets. A person who has fallen and is in pain should not be moved because movement may displace the bone and cause further damage. If a neck injury is suspected, the head should be kept very still.

If possible, gently cover any obvious wounds with dressings. Stop bleeding with direct pressure.

Do not give food or drink. This could delay surgery if an anesthetic is needed.

PAIN THAT IS MORE THAN A MINOR DISCOMFORT

Pains in the chest, arms, or jaw, or dizziness and nausea can be serious. Seniors should stop exercising at once and consult a doctor. A pain is probably serious if it wakes you up at night. See a doctor about it.

MINOR ACHES AND PAINS AND MINOR INJURIES

Soreness. We can expect sore muscles and stiffness when we first exercise or after a break. The pain will go away in a few days. Just remember to do everything in moderation. Mild discomfort is normal.

If you over exercise you may experience DOMS, which you will find in the glossary as standing for "Delayed Onset of Muscle Soreness." The fact that trainers use initials for this tells you a little about its frequency.

This is soreness that lasts from forty-eight to seventy-two hours after exercising. Stretching exercises and drinking plenty of water help prevent this soreness. Depending upon the severity, one source suggests the way to treat DOMS is to do the same exercise the next day but less intensely.

INVOLUNTARY MUSCLE CONTRACTIONS

Involuntary muscle contractions follow a progression of seriousness.

Twitching. The twitches come and go and are irritating but not painful or serious.

Spasm. This is more serious and may happen by overstretching or in the presence of an injury. The muscles go into spasm to "protect" the injured body part. The pain can be intense. A spasm has the potential to impede blood flow and can hinder, but does not prevent, function.

A muscle cramp. This is the most intense and painful involuntary muscle contraction. It is sufficiently intense to stop circulation as well as all functional use.

A muscle cramp occurs when a muscle involuntarily contracts so strongly that it impedes blood flow. The cause can be dehydration (not getting enough water when we exercise), diuretics, or straining the muscle by over exercising.

Treatment of a Cramp. A cold pack will relax the tense muscles. But more immediate methods also exist. Attempt to stretch the cramping muscle in any safe position you are able.

Once the cramp releases, massage the affected area. The main thing is to increase the blood flow.

For an arm cramp, hold your elbow and bend your arm back and forth. For a foot cramp, pull up on the toes.

For a calf cramp, put your weight on the cramped leg and slightly bend your knee. If this doesn't help, hold the ball of your foot and pull toward the knee cap.

For a hamstring cramp, keep both legs straight and lean forward at the waist.

If you're awakened with a cramp in the calf, bend your toes and foot upward, toward your knees, or stretch the heel cord.

If it's a thigh cramp, the best thing you can do is massage. Once the cramp releases, walking may be painful for a while but helpful in time.

If you have frequent cramps, see your doctor. Options are prescribed muscle relaxers, stretching exercises, and/or plenty of water.

MUSCLE STRAINS

A strain can happen because of overextending a muscle or tendon. You are most likely to get these in the lower back or thigh (hamstrings and quadriceps) and can last for several months.

They commonly occur when you over exercise, but they may be the result of trauma. The pain is directly over the strained muscle.

If the strain is serious enough to keep you from going about your daily routines, see a doctor. If it is intense pain, especially after a fall, it could be a fracture and should be X-rayed.

A BASIC TREATMENT: RICE PLUS ASPIRIN

The standard treatment for an ordinary strain has always been RICE. Now some sports medicine types make it PRICE.

P= protection
R= rest
I= icing
C= compression
E= elevation

The *P* stands for protection in the form of a wrap, cast, brace, crutches, etc. We're not sure this addition to the acronym will catch on.

The *R* stands for rest, generally for at least twenty-four hours. This includes not putting any further strain on the injury too soon by exercising or walking.

The *I* is for ice. This reduces inflammation. When you remove the ice, the blood rushes back in. Apply ice for thirty minutes immediately after an injury and later several times a day for twenty to thirty minutes. Continue icing for twenty-four to seventy-two hours if necessary.

The *C* is for compression to hold down swelling (with bandages or elastic wraps).

The *E* is for elevation above the level of your heart. This helps reduce swelling.

Anti-inflammatory drugs may be an option but may be contraindicated in the presence of bleeding. Check with you doctor.

Why Heat and Cold Packs Are So Helpful

After forty-eight to seventy-two hours, some suggest we switch to heat, though this is debatable. One study found that continued icing at twenty-minute intervals worked better than heat. So try both and continue the one that works.

Cold numbs nerves and so lessens the pain. It also reduces inflammation by shrinking the blood vessels around the injury. If you have arthritis in your feet where blood vessels are already narrow, avoid cold packs.

Reusable cold packs are pliable and refreeze quickly, or you can use packages of frozen peas or corn as long as you label them "don't eat" when they are returned to the freezer.

Heat increases the blood flow and is good for chronic pain and to reduce stiffness. Moist heat may be more effective since it also seems to promote relaxation.

Heat wraps maintain a steady temperature of 104 degrees to reduce minor pain and stiffness. Some of the products offered are Therma Care Air-Activated Heat Wrap, Beyond BodiHeat, and Grabber My Coal Body Warmer.

Don reports that the hot moist packs he uses in physical therapy begin to cool after twenty to thirty minutes. The skin will redden after each application, and they can be used several times a day providing the body part has a chance to cool to normal temperatures. Beware that prolonged use of heat overtime will discolor the skin.

An electric heating pad will maintain the heat and temperature you indicate but will burn if left on too long. The body must dissipate any heat above that of the body temperature, and there is a limit on how long it can do this.

Those who have had knee replacements should remember that the metal of the replacement can get very hot and cause surface burns if you put a heating pad over it too long. I prefer the use of cold since edema reduction is often desired.

Sprains

These happen when we overstretch or tear ligaments. They often occur in the ankle or knee making it difficult to walk. A simple ankle or knee sprain takes about a month to heal.

Coaches used to recommend that players "just walk it off." PRICE (which emphasizes rest) is the treatment now preferred. Ligaments heal slowly and reinjuring just prolongs the recovery time.

Dr. Bruce Beynnon, a biomechanical engineer at the University of Vermont, and colleagues found a difference in patterns in the sprains of men and women. Women'=s risks are related to balance and lack of strength in opposing muscle groups, a problem we will deal with shortly. Sprains for men were found to be more the result of the restricted range of motion in the joint.

Shin Splints

These are less likely to occur for unsteady Seniors since jumping, running, or jogging on hard surfaces causes them. Microtears in the leg muscles occur where the muscle attaches to the bone resulting in inflammation. The standard treatment again is RICE.

STITCHES

These sharp pains in your side sometimes happen while you exercise. You need to bend forward and tighten your abdomen while you breathe deeply and purse your lips. You also could tighten your belt. Or you can try raising your hands over your head.

ACHILLES TENDINITIS

The Achilles tendon connects the calf muscles to the heel and becomes inflamed. If left untreated, scar tissue may develop as well as chronic pain and impaired gait. Again, PRICE.

MUSCLES OUT OF BALANCE

This occurs when one muscle becomes stronger that the opposing muscle. It can happen if we go overboard on one kind of exercise. A personal trainer or a physical therapist will be able to identify this and get you back on the right track.

Women tend to have stronger quads (front of thigh) than hamstrings (back of thigh), perhaps from walking in high heels. This can lead to hamstring strains, sprains, or knee injuries and the researchers find that women do get more knee injuries than men do.

BUILDUP OF LACTIC ACID

You may have been warned that over exercising results in over production of lactic acid. It has long been thought that this causes stiffness and pain in the legs. This notion was based on studies a Nobel laureate made in the early 1900s.

More recently, George A. Brooks of the Department of Integrative Biology at the University of California, Berkeley, found that lactic acid is actually an energy source, helpful to those athletes who push themselves to their limit and then use it to get an extra burst of energy. He says of the previous theory, "It's one of the classic mistakes in the history of science."

So the experts flip-flop, and we progress.

POLAR BEAR POOLS

Fitness centers and health clubs have polar bear pools on the theory that when you sit in one for a while, the blood leaves your legs. When you get out and get into a warm relaxation pool, the blood flows back into your limbs. This is supposed to have a healing effect on tired muscles after exercising.

This is not recommended for those with heart problems or weak will power.

MEDICATIONS TO CONTROL PAIN AND STIFFNESS

NSAIDs (Nonsteroidal Anti-inflammatory Drugs). These drugs decrease the production of substances that send pain messages to the brain (prostaglandins) as well as reduce inflammation and stiffness. Over twenty-five now exist. Several are available over the counter for arthritics.

But they unfortunately have side effects. Taken regularly, they may cause stomach bleeding. Ibuprofen was thought to be the least hard on the stomach, but a 2005 study at McMasters University in Ontario warns against daily use of high doses of ibuprofen 400 mg or more per day. All except aspirin may also cause an increased risk of cardiovascular problems, heart attacks, or strokes.

Aspirin. This old standby reduces inflammation and is also a blood thinner. It is hard on stomach but effective for aches, stiffness, and pain. Regular use increases the risk of high blood pressure.

Many doctors recommend taking a baby aspirin every day to protect your heart and thin your blood. Check with *your* doctor first.

Stomach-protecting drugs. Doctors recommend two stomach-protecting drugs to be taken to offset the effects of NSAIDs on the stomach

The first are known as H2 receptor antagonists—Tagament, Zantac, Axid, and Pepsid A. C.

More recently, researchers have developed a second type of stomach-protecting drug called proton pump inhibitors—Prilosec, Nexium, Prevacid, and Protonix.

Again, we are warned against overuse.

It also may help our digestion if we keep our mouth closed when drinking or eating so we don't swallow air. Also, the experts suggest that we not take another bite until we've swallowed the last one. And as our mothers used to say, we must chew our food well so we don't become a client for one of those CPR types just looking around for someone to practice on.

Acetaminophen. This is not an NSAID. The main over-the-counter drug is Tylenol, though discount stores may sell the drug cheaper as acetaminophen. It does not increase the risk of high blood pressure.

Physicians recommend no more than 4,000 mg a day (four grams) since overdosing is the most common cause of acute liver damage. Just doubling the maximum daily dose can be enough to kill.

The company that makes Tylenol advertises: "If you're not going to read the label, don't buy our product."

Dr. William Lee of the University of Texas Southwestern Medical Center and Dr. Anne Larsen of the University of Washington Medical Center made a study of 662 cases of acute liver failure attributed to acetaminophen. Some 44 percent were the result of suicide attempts (you can't blame the drug for that), but 48 percent were from unintentional overdoses; the other 8 percent were from unknown causes.

The problem is that acetaminophen is also a part of a number of over-the-counter remedies such as Excedrin, Nyquill Cold/Flu, or Theraflu. Sometimes this information is not noted on the package. It is also part of some prescription narcotics. (Sixty-three percent of the unintentional overdoses fit this category.)

Sweet cherries. Michigan raises a good many sweet cherries for export. The researchers at Michigan State University tested and found that cherries were as effective in treating pain and stiffness as most NSAIDs. As far as we know, this study has not been replicated elsewhere.

Methylsulfonylmethane (MSM). This drug, in trials, has shown moderate improvement for pain for those with osteoarthritis.

Glucosamine Chondroitin. The National Institutes of Health in 2006 reported on a study they had funded—the largest study yet done of glucosamine's effect on arthritis. It involved 1,538 patients at sixteen medical centers. They found chondroitin had little effect while glucosamine was effective for about 20 percent who used it or one in five. It has most effect on the moderate to severe cases of arthritis.

Drug safety. The U.S. Food and Drug Administration's website to help consumers learn about the risks of prescription and over-the-counter drugs is www.fda.gov/dcer (Click the box "Drug Safety.")

SALVES, CREAMS, AND OINTMENTS (TOPICAL ANALGESICS)

Analgesic is the fancy name for pain killer. With the news about the digestive problems that are the side effects of NSAIDs, some Seniors are turning at least part of the time to over-the-counter creams, salves, ointments, balms, sticks, or patches.

These products do not kill the pain but distract by creating temporary sensations of warmth or coolness. They can be either hot or cold, and a few are both.

They are helpful for only short-term relief and won't ease all joint pain, but you may decide that's good enough. To maintain their effect, these products must be used four to five times a day.

The choices. The cooling salves contain such ingredients as menthol, camphor, or wintergreen oil. The deep heat salves generally contain salicylates, the major ingredient in aspirin, and may interact negatively with blood thinners such as warfarin.

The salves that contain capsaicin (Zostrix, Capzasin), have the ingredient that makes hot peppers so hot. These deaden the nerve endings that send pain signals to the brain. It takes at least a week or two of use for three or four times a day before this deadening takes effect and has to be continued to keep the pain deadened. Some Seniors decide not to use this salve because of the burning sensation that results from continued use.

After use of any salve, hands should be washed, and we should avoid touching the face, children, or pets. This is especially true of capsaicin since it can burn on contact.

Numbing patches. These contain a local anesthetic. You can only obtain them with a prescription. They are used on flat surfaces and should be changed twice a day. The main ingredient of the lidocaine patches is lidoderm.

NSAID creams and lotions. These have been used in Canada and Europe, but only one is available for general use in the United States as we write. This is Solarze, prescribed for skin problems. The NSAID used is diclofenac. More may be approved.

Iboprofin cream and diclofenac lotion are available in Canada by prescription and over-the-counter in England.

OTHER METHODS TO CONTROL PAIN

Homeopathic remedies. Homeopathic medicine is based on the philosophy that the body is capable of healing itself. Its origin is over two hundred years old and comes from the idea that "like causes like." In short, a substance that causes a symptom in a healthy person can also be the cure when reintroduced in minute quantities.

Homeopathic remedies are derived from substances that come from plants, minerals, or minerals. The U.S. Food and Drug Administration (FDA) regulates the homeopathic practice but does not evaluate the remedies for safety or effectiveness.

Considering the number of patients who claim homeopathy works suggests that vigorous clinical research is warranted to give it credibility in the medical profession. However, drug companies fund much of that research and have little to gain and much to lose if homeopathic claims are validated.

Regrettably, medical practice guidelines may discourage physicians from even recommending homeopathic remedies. Good luck!

Cognitive Behavioral Therapy (CBT). This is a therapeutic treatment that through a series of exercises, causes us to emphasize positive thoughts and eliminate the you know what.

They say we can replace our physical pains with lesser pains as a distraction. One way, we suggest, is to buy a computer for its aggravation effect. Just kidding!

Guided imagery. We are told to think of happy times, like the time we put a nickel in the slot machine and hit the jackpot and got a Mickey Mouse watch or of the day we woke up to look out at our backyard and saw the beauty of a snowfall (banish all thoughts about the driveway). Some people imagine their muscles melting. Anyhow, relax!

Hypnosis. Some physicians use this technique. Contrary to popular misconceptions, the subject is aware of what is happening and cannot be caused to do things contrary to his or her own desires. The procedure is safe and has few side effects when an expert does the hypnotizing.

Meditation and Mindfulness. One form of meditation is to repeat a phrase over and over, thus clearing the mind of anxieties and also, it is found, the feeling of pain.

The May-June issue 2006 of *Arthritis Today* of the Arthritis Foundation describes a second technique called mindfulness. This is essentially becoming intensely aware of things about us. For example, when we brush our teeth, we become very aware of the toothpaste oozing out of the tube, the mint taste of the toothpaste, the sound and feel of the brushing on teeth and fingers, and the wetness and coolness of water when you flush your mouth. Also, you notice your posture and watch the water disappear down the drain, etc.

This can't do any harm and it may help. It can only make us appreciate more the beauty and wonder of God's good green Earth. It may even turn us into poets.

OTHER MEDICATIONS FOR SPECIFIC PROBLEMS

Calcium. It is necessary to strengthen bones (1200 mg a day recommended). But note that we get some in our multivitamins and in milk. Another factor is if the calcium being ingested is being absorbed. It's complicated but worth checking out.

Fosomax, Actonel, and Boniva. Prescribed drugs used to increase bone density. Read the negative side effects carefully and check with your doctor.

Cod liver oil. It was found to delay cartilage damage as well as lowering heart disease risk but not generally recommended today because of potentially toxic doses of vitamins A and D.

Multivitamins. We Seniors are advised to gulp down a multi every day. To reduce the risk of heart disease, it should contain at least 400 mcg (micrograms) of folic acid, 3 mg of B6, and 2 mg of B12. We should add that now some researchers question the effectiveness of multivitamins.

Vitamin D (The Sunshine Vitamin). It keeps bones strong, which helps prevent falls and breaks if you do fall. Your multivitamins should contain 400 IU. We also get vitamin D from other sources such as the sun, milk, fortified breakfast foods, and cold-water fish such as mackerel, salmon, and sardines.

Researchers now recommend 800 IU for Seniors, and some think it should be 1,000 mg. Those of us in northern climates may want to consider this supplement in winter.

Some researchers are also theorizing that vitamin D may improve balance, presumably because it strengthens our rickety bones.

Miracle supplements. Go easy on these. Let's save our money so we can get in on the ground floor the next time some stranger approaches us with the news that the Brooklyn Bridge out there in New York City is again up for sale. We may even be able to buy in for a piece of that Alaska Bridge to nowhere. No use wasting it on miracle supplements.

Charlie tries a miracle treatment. A woman wrote into one of those medical columns in the newspaper saying she found that smearing Vicks Vapo Rub on her legs helped reduce her peripheral neuropathy. He looked at the Vicks label on a jar and found it contained camphor and menthol, both of which might stir up nerve endings, as well as eucalyptus. It seemed harmless, so he tried it.

Don said if something doesn't work after a month to six weeks, it probably will never work. It didn't work for Charlie, and he thinks it's nice to no longer smell like he has a bad cough, so people shy away when he sits down next to them.

Just for the record, Charlie says he would never embrace any kooky treatment that asked him to swallow some concoction, no matter what it promised. For that, he wants a doctor's prescription or assurances from a reliable source that it's not harmful and has no side effects. What are the chances of that? And he checks labels before smearing stuff on his leg.

Side Effects from Drug Interactions

The National Council on Aging has coproduced a website on the risk of mixing over-the-counter and prescription medicines at *www.senior-med-safety.com.*

Talking Prescription Bottles

This is the latest for those of us Seniors who have trouble figuring out what the prescription tacked on the bottle means. We just press a button and listen.

Drug Instruction Inserts

The Food and Drug Administration (FDA) has made new rules for those inserts that come folded up with drugs and generally go on for pages of tiny print. They are requiring the manufacturers of new drugs to include a section of highlights that will tell us the drug's risks and benefits. A contents section will also be added.

Decoding Our Doctor's Prescription Forms

Most of us may have wondered what those doctor notations mean, assuming we can puzzle out the writing. Maybe the *Reader's Digest* was being mischievous. In their March 2006 issue, they let us in on our doctor's secret code. Here it is.

ac	before meals
alt die	alternate days
bid	twice a day
c̄	(with a line above the c) with
dol urg	when pain is severe
hs	at
prn	when needed

sig	write on label
sos	if necessary
stat	immediately
tid	three times a day
2X	refill two times

"Common Injuries Treatment and Medications" What Was That Chapter All About?

If you fall, check first for pain before trying to get up. If you suspect a serious injury, call 911 for paramedic, and don't let yourself be moved. Ask for blankets to keep warm and don't take food or drink.

Treatment is described for minor injuries such as soreness, twitches, spasms, cramps, sprains, strains, and stitches. Use RICE or PRICE. Muscle balance and lactic acid, heat and cold packs, and polar bear pools are discussed as well as medications such as aspirin, NSAIDs, stomach-protecting drugs, acetaminophen, and MSM.

Glucosamine Chondroitin is reviewed as well as such topical analgesics as salves, creams, ointments, and numbing patches.

Homeopathic remedies, Cognitive Behavioral Therapy (CBT), Guided imagery, hypnosis. meditation and mindfulness are pain reducing techniques used by some.

Where to go to find out about side effects from drug interactions, drug inserts, and how to decode your doctor's prescription are discussed.

Chapter 41

DIET AND WEIGHT

No sermon needed here. We know, we know.

Physicians emphasize the relationship of weight to diabetes and cardiovascular problems. But for us, it's also what extra weight does to our knees. Being heavy also makes it more difficult to exercise, in part because you are soon out of breath.

A study at Wake Forest University found that during a one-mile walk, every pound of weight adds an additional 4,800 pounds of load on the knees. The lesson unsteady Seniors are supposed to get from this interesting fact is not that we should avoid one-mile walks but something else.

LOOSE WRISTWATCHES

After we have been exercising a while, we may notice that our wristwatch has slipped around our wrist. The physical therapists tell us that, even so, the scale may not show a weight loss. That's because some of the stored fat has been used for fueling the exercises. How about that!

OUR METABOLIC RATE

Our metabolism determines how the food we consume gets changed into fuel for activity, tissue repair, and storage. With less activity, more calories go into storage, generally around our waists and hips.

Our metabolic rate goes down as we get older and less active. But we'll only gain weight if we absorb as many pizzas and milkshakes as we did when we unsteady Seniors were carefree high schoolers. At least so say we know who.

When we exercise, it not only reduces the fat content in the muscles, it also strengthens the muscles. A well-conditioned muscle will in turn burn more calories even at rest. This will increase the basal metabolic rate. The end result is fewer calories going into storage.

MEASURES OF CORRECT WEIGHT

Maybe just looking at what the scale tells us is enough, but the experts have devised other measures.

Belt size. A rough measure for determining overweight is our belt size. For males, we're overweight if the belt size is forty inches or above; for females, it's thirty-five inches or above. However, this measure isn't foolproof because it doesn't take height into account.

The BMI (Body-Mass Index). The BMI has been the standard way of determining ideal weight. It is the basis for all those weight charts we come across.

We divide our weight in pounds by our height in inches squared. Then multiply by 703. We're overweight if the result is 25 to 29.9. Those who are obese have a rate over 30. A government website will compute your BMI for you at *www.nhlbisupport.com/bmi.*

Like all measures, the BMI has problems. One is that muscle weight is treated the same as fat. And it doesn't indicate where excess fat is carried in the body. Belly fat is a greater health risk than fat around the hips or bottom.

Waist-to-hip measure. British researchers have found that for those of us over seventy-five a better measure is that found by dividing waist measure by hip measure. Those who have a result that is close 1.0 are more likely to be at risk for disease later on than those with a result closer to 0.8.

FAT BUT FIT

A recent study suggests that exercise may offset some of the bad effects of being overweight, what they call being "fat but fit." The study suggests that death rates for males who are "fat but fit" are less than those who are "lean but unfit" (sedentary). "Fat but fit" women had the same death rates as "lean but unfit." You women already know that the world isn't fair.

The problem is that someone who is fat is less likely to exercise enough to also qualify as being fit as well as fat. But that won't include us anymore.

A little overweight. Latest research, published in the *Journal of the American Medical Association*, goes a little further, leaving out the exercise. It suggests that those who are slightly overweight live longer than the very thin or those grossly overweight.

The theory is that those who are a little overweight have some stored-up energy to use if they get sick. This is an example when a little is good and more is not. Being grossly overweight is not healthy and puts one in danger of other complications. If a little overweight is confirmed in other studies we may see some changes in the kinds of advice on weight that the experts hand out.

That study only covered seven years. Critics suggest that may not have been a long-enough period for heart problems to show up in the slightly overweight.

WHAT WE EAT

We could use Mr. Wither's advice, the fellow who's still biking around at eighty-six—avoid foods loaded with trans fats, hydrogenated fats, partially hydrogenated fats, and sodium. Concentrate on fruits and vegetables.

Some would also add eat fish more frequently than beef or pork. The omega-3 fatty acids are good for you. A snack of a handful of nuts is also recommended. Go easy on commercially baked foods and those tasty chip products.

Here are other advice generously given by experts.

Keep servings small. Don't take seconds. Eat only one peanut at a time and chew and swallow it before you grab another.

Some experts even suggest we eat TV dinners because the portions are fixed; however, they are apt to be full of sodium. What we know for sure is that eating out in restaurants doesn't lead to weight loss.

The Tony Martin Plan. That crooner of World War II days, Tony Martin, who was still doing an occasional five-night singing gig at age ninety-five, said he's lived so long and stayed active in part because he ate only two meals a day. He claimed he weighed in the 160s, and he was married to Cyd Charisse too, in case you're interested.

Measuring portions. If you get so serious about dieting that you measure portions, here is something to help you out.

One cup of cereal = a fist
Half a cup of cooked rice, pasta, or potato = half a baseball
One medium fruit = a baseball
One and a half ounces of low fat or fat free cheese = four stacked dice
Two tablespoons of peanut butter = a Ping-Pong ball
Three ounces of meat or poultry = a deck of cards

WHAT WE DRINK

The experts still haven't heard about anything much better to drink than water.

Consider colas: They have no nutritional value, are heavy in sugar, and contain needless calories. Diet colas, on the other hand, produce an accumulated toxic effect on our system.

The caffeine in soft drinks and tea and coffee is a diuretic. Insufficient hydration promotes muscle cramps. Power drinks are heavy in calories.

WHERE IT'S ALL HEADING

Those of us Seniors who have watched the antismoking campaign as it unfolded can see the direction in which the nation is going on the topic of weight.

A November 3, 2005 news item was headed "Supermodel Finds Out It's Not Fun to Be Fat." Tyra Banks, a TV show host, decided to wear a fat suit to find out how it felt to be grossly overweight.

She reported, "I started walking down the street, and, within 10 seconds, a trio of people looked at me, snickered, looked me right in my eye, and started pointing and laughing in my face. I had no idea it was that blatant."

So we've all been warned.

Less weight is easier on the knees. A smaller belly will also keep our center of gravity more over our feet. The result is better balance.

That's all you get here. Plenty of weight loss books exist that go into great detail on the latest weight loss fad diet.

What Was That Chapter All About?

For unsteady Seniors, a major aspect of being overweight is the pressure it puts on our knees. Our metabolism rate determines the calories we store. Exercise raises the metabolism rate and burns calories. Several ways have been developed for measuring our desirable weight. All have critics.

The fat-but-fit argument is reviewed as well as whether being slightly overweight is a health advantage. Good eating habits are briefly noted.

Chapter 42

Interpreting Research Results

Don said when he read this chapter, prepared mainly by Charlie, "You brought something to my mind that I heard many times from my pathology professor at the Mayo Clinic. He stressed that the *Reader's Digest* is not a medical journal. Yet the public gets their medical information from it, reading the newspapers, good housekeeping, etc., where the criteria for publishing is not the same as is in medical journals. The problem is that too often we are told what to believe with little scientific basis."

So beware of media hype and ballyhoo.

How Medical Researchers Make a Finding

First, remember that a single study of whatever kind is only an indication. Researchers are prudent. They want many studies that come to the same finding before they are willing to accept it.

They also want the findings to be reported as specific to the group studied. It was women researchers who pointed out that many of the findings that were done with a male sample did not necessarily apply to women.

Also, researchers have to be careful not to endanger the life or health of subjects. They can't keep a known cure from those in their experiment. Uncertainty about side effects makes it difficult to include pregnant women or young children in many studies.

Types of Research Studies

The two types of research studies are those examining relationships and those of controlled experiments. The first is suggestive of an association between two items; the second attempts to confirm that one caused the other.

Relationship Studies

These studies show a statistical relationship between two variables, for example between reduction in pain for people who were arthritic and eating cherries for breakfast.

Epidemiological studies are relationship studies in the health field. They deal with a disease and characteristics or traits associated with its occurrence.

If a relationship is found, it does not prove that one item caused the other since a third or more variables might bring about the relationship. Say disease X is associated with eating a certain kind of fruit. Perhaps it was something they sprayed on the fruit to preserve it that caused the relationship.

Any relationship found can only be confirmed in a series of controlled clinical experiments, though this isn't always possible.

Relationship studies sometimes ask persons to remember what they did in the past and clearly these are not wholly reliable.

This is why the reports of studies of relationships often use the word "may" to describe their findings. "May" does not mean "this is a cause." It only means maybe.

Still, when a relationship is shown over and over, such relationship studies can be so strong statistically as to be interpreted as causal, as for example the relationship between smoking and lung cancer.

Untestable relationships. Some relationships that are found cannot be tested or can only be tested with great difficulty or great expense. The lung cancer-smoking relationship is an example impossible to test in a lab experiment except on mice.

Back at the time of the Spanish American War, the researchers suspected the bite of an infected mosquito transmitted yellow fever.

They experimented on volunteers and on themselves, with sometimes disastrous results, including some deaths. That kind of experiment would not be permitted today.

So we may sometimes have to settle for relationship studies and repeat the study many times with different population groups. Statisticians then work out a number to show the probability that the relationship is genuine and did not occur by chance.

Pseudorelationships. Professors of statistics are fond of demonstrating that pseudo-relationships do occur. For example, and I'm making this up, they might discover a statistically significant relationship between the rainfall in Burma and the divorce rate in Utah—a relationship that is only a coincidence, but such pseudorelationships do pop up.

Observational studies. These are a form of relationship study in which a group is studied over time. If a subgroup can be isolated, say those that over the course of years develop rheumatoid arthritis, researchers try to determine whether members of this group have common traits that are found less frequently or not at all in the rest of the study group.

The value of relationship studies. These studies give us hints of possible causes of certain effects, causes that perhaps can later be tested in a laboratory in a controlled double-blind experiment.

DOUBLE-BLIND CLINICAL TESTS

These are experimental studies that attempt to tie a specific agent (the cause) to a specific outcome (the effect). If done under controlled conditions, they are considered the most reliable findings.

Two groups are used to test the effect of a new drug. The researchers may study those who share a common characteristic (those who have severe arthritis pains) or they choose from the general population, selected at random if, say theoretically, it is a drug to raise everyone's IQ to 200.

Part of the group is given the drug; the rest, called the control group, is given a placebo, a harmless substance that looks like, but is not, the drug. The subjects must be assigned randomly to each group.

The blind part first off is that the subjects do not know which group they are in. The experiment is double blind if the experimenters themselves don't know who is in either group until the experiment is complete and the findings are tabulated.

A crucial step is analysis of the findings. Note that a negative finding, that is that no relationship exists, may sometimes be important, for example the study already cited on glucosamine.

The results are tested statistically to determine if the differences we find between the two groups are greater than what would occur by chance, that it is a statistically significant relationship.

Clinical trials of drugs that are marketed must be approved ahead of time by the FDA. The drug must first be tested on animals before the manufacturer asks the FDA for permission to test on humans. The experiment is reviewed by an independent group of experts. The researchers also look for possible side effects.

Note that many of these tests could not easily be done in a relationship study since giving people a drug over a period of years may be too costly or too dangerous.

Many of these experimental trials are time consuming, and so the experimenting agency may legitimately pay the volunteers. This may be the easiest way to recruit those having a specific condition that the medication hopes to ameliorate. And the researchers themselves are often underwritten by the drug company. Yet often no one else would have the interest to finance such a study. All of this may raise problems concerning the results found.

Cumulative studies. A single successful double-blind experiment is also not sufficient. Others must be able to do the same study and get the same results. A study in Japan may get different results than a study made in Sweden for reasons not immediately apparent but having something to do with the different ethnic populations.

Sooner or later, researchers will gather together all the studies of a similar problem, pick out only those that follow defensible procedures, question the far out findings, and reject those studies flawed in some respect. They then report the common conclusions reached. If there are many different results, it's back to the drawing board. Now you know why experts sometimes exchange their minds.

JUDGING STUDIES

When we read about reports of studies in a newspaper, our best guide to quality is who did the study and where it was published.

Was it done at a major university or medical school? Was it published in a peer-reviewed journal such as the *New England Journal of Medicine*, where we know other scientists in the field have reviewed the procedures used? Was it the journal of a recognized professional association?

We are at the mercy of the professionalism of the researcher, which, as laymen, is probably our best and only guide to the value of a finding.

A FLAWED EXPERIMENT

So here's a quick test. Listening to the tape of an old *Bob Hope* show while exercising, I heard the announcer tout a test probably suggested by the ads that asked, "Which twin is wearing the Tony?"

The test on the *Hope* show was also of twins. One was given Pepsodent to brush her teeth with and the other "another product." After three months, it was reported that the girl who used Pepsodent had whiter teeth.

We get no information how whiteness was measured or whether the other product was made out of street sweepings. Were the twins paid? Now how could this wonderful experiment be improved?

You got it. The twins knew who was paying them to take the test, and they knew what result was hoped for. Pepsodent seems to have made no effort to make this a double-blind experiment. The twins should not have known whether they were using Pepsodent or that obviously inferior other product. Maybe those who used Pepsodent brushed harder and oftener and those who used the other product persuaded themselves it tasted like wallpaper paste and didn't brush.

And we get a sample of two. Statisticians generally like at least thirty cases. Sometimes this isn't possible. Beer manufacturers needed to test product quality of batches of their bottled product more economically than opening half of each batch. They developed what is called small-sample statistics, but even these depend on more than two cases.

When you hear a product advertised as "acts twice as fast," ask, "acts twice as fast as what—a gum drop?"

THE SECRET STATISTIC DOCTORS USE

Suppose we had a test of a drug, five thousand take the drug and five thousand take a placebo. Then we test for the numbers in each group that developed a cold in the next month. It is reported that twice as many persons in the placebo group had a cold than did those taking the cold-fighting drug.

Sounds like a pretty impressive finding?

But suppose in this study of five thousand, only three persons in all turned up with a cold that month. Two were in the placebo group and only one in the drug taking group. It's now less impressive since this might just be a coincidence.

Doctors thus want to know another statistic called NNT which stands for "Number Needed to Treat." The NNT for this study would be 2,500 since 5,000 had to take the drug to prevent two colds.

If the test had been of a cold-fighting drug with possible or known side effects, the doctor might further question whether it was worth prescribing the drug with only one in 2,500 benefitting and the possible risk of complications (two cases for 5000 subjects.) The NNT is not generally given for most studies. The physician simply decides whether the drug's success rate plus the possible risk of a negative side effect makes it worth prescribing.

WHAT WAS THAT CHAPTER ALL ABOUT?

Relationship studies with their value and drawbacks. Double-blind experimental studies. How we can, as laymen, judge findings? An example was given of a flawed experiment and the NNT.

Chapter 43

A Glossary of Terms

(so we unsteady Seniors can

understand the experts)

Abs. The abdominal muscles.

Abds. Abductors are the muscles of the outer shoulders and hips.

Abduction. Movements away from the body.

Adds. Adductors are the muscles of the inner thighs.

Adduction. Sideway movements toward the body.

Aerobic or endurance training. Exercises that strengthen the heart and burn calories.

Biceps. Muscles to the front of the upper arm.

BMI. Body Mass Index determines ideal body weight. See chapter on diet to find out how to calculate.

BMR. Basal Metabolic Rate (BMR) or sometimes called Resting Metabolic Rate (RMR) is the number of calories our bodies burn each day at rest—that is the number of calories we need just to keep us going.

Circuit training. A circuit of exercises done one after the other, often on a series of machines that manufacturers have designed to work all muscle groupings.

Core muscles. The core muscles Joseph H. Pilates zeroed in on are the band of about 29 muscles that encircle the torso-hips, pelvis, spine, and abdomen. Pilates believed that strengthening these core muscles would stabilize the spine and pelvis and would lead to a better transfer of power to the extremities-the legs, arms, and shoulders. He argued this would lead to fewer injuries and to less frequent and intense lower back pain. Today neurologists are suggesting that this may also help with the balance problems faced by Seniors.

Cross-training. Refers to the training in one type of activity in order to gain proficiency in another. For balance-challenged Seniors, they may get conditioned on a recumbent bike in an effort to improve their lower extremity strength for walking.

Density training. Taking less time between sets at the beginning of the workout when the muscles aren't tired and more time toward the end of the workout.

DOMS. Delayed Onset of Muscle Soreness. This soreness occurs forty-eight to seventy-two hours after exercising, not just the next morning. Stretching exercises and drinking plenty of water help prevent DOMS.

Endorphins and Enkephalins. These are the natural narcotics released into our systems as a direct result of aerobic exercises. In addition to being natural pain relievers, they also are mood elevators (makes us feel good).

Extension. Straightening, as an arm or leg.

Fascia. A thin layer of tissue that covers, supports, or binds together a muscle, part, or organ.

Flex. Bend, as an arm or leg.

Flexibility. The pliability of muscles and joints.

Gluteals. Also called glutes; are the three muscles at our buttocks.

Hamstrings. Sometimes called hams or hammys (ugh!) are located behind the thighs. Tight hamstrings may contribute to lower back pain.

Handbook. A guide that tries to inform you about all the practical things you should know about a subject. It is designed to be consulted later as a reference.

Isometric exercises. Contraction of muscles without movement of what may be painful joints.

Isotonic exercises. The resistance used is gravity.

Joints. Found where two bones come together. The joints are where we find the cushioning that keeps bones from rubbing together and thus allows us to move our limbs, etc.

Ligaments. Connective tissue that connect bones to each other.

Metabolism. The rate at which digested fats, proteins, and carbohydrates mix with oxygen and are burned to create energy. The excess may be used for repair but more likely is stored as fat and results in weight gain. Our metabolism declines with age.

Muscle. Muscles are the thick fibrous tissues that contract and expand to allow movement around joints. In an eccentric contraction, the muscle elongates as it contracts. For example, hold a weight in your hand with the elbow flexed to ninety degrees. As you lower the weight, the biceps contract to control the rate of descent but elongates at the same time.

Muscle cramps. Extremely painful and may stop circulation as well as functional use. These involuntary contractions may occur in the extremities or abdomen.

Muscle spasm. Associated with pain with the potential to impede blood flow but does not prevent function. They usually occur to protect a body part after injury.

Muscle strains. The pain from overextending a muscle. It is most likely to occur in the lower back or thigh (hamstrings and quadriceps).

NSAIDs. Nonsteroidal Anti-inflammatory Drugs taken to lessen the pain and stiffness of arthritis. They do not, however, slow the disease.

Orthotics. Ankle or knee braces and shoe inserts.

Placebo. To make certain an experiment is blind so far as the participants or the researchers know, one group is given the experimental drug and the other a harmless substance, a placebo, that looks like the drug.

Placebo effect. Sometimes just being part of the experiment causes improvement, even though the participant has only received a placebo.

Postural stability. A more precise word for steadiness and balance.

Proprioception or position sense. Recognizing where our arms, hands, legs, and feet are without looking.

Quads. The quadriceps are the four muscles front of the thighs.

Range of motion (ROM). The available movement of a body part at a specific joint. For example, how much can we bend the forearm at the elbow or how far we can extend the leg at the knee.

Reps (Repetitions). The number of times we do an exercise.

Resistance, Weight, or Strength training. Exercises that use gravity or other resistance to challenge muscles.

RMR. Resting metabolism rate.

ROM. Range of motion.

Sets. A group of repetitions of an exercise. A rest period separates sets.

Sprain. What may happen when we overstretch or partially tear ligaments.

Stepping stones. Insights in why we do what we do to recover balance.

Stretching, flexibility, or Range of motion exercises. Movement of joints to increase circulation to reduce stiffness and bend an arm, leg, or toe to its farthest extent.

Tendons. Tendons attach muscles to bones. Tendinitis occurs when we inflame the tendons through an injury or overuse.

Stretch bands. Those five-inch-wide, rubberish, elastic bands. They come from two feet to a yard or so long. The different colors indicate the level of resistance.

Triceps. Muscles in the back of the upper arm.

Twitch. A non-sustained involuntary muscle contraction. These are usually more irritating than painful.

Twitching. An exercise in which voluntary isometric contractions of muscles around a painful joint occur without moving the joint.

PART FOUR

Chapter 44

QUESTIONS UNSTEADY
SENIORS ASK US

Does the weather affect our balancing? Yes, a lot of people think so, especially when a front goes through.

Can our balance vary from day to day? Yes. Some days we wake up with the old aches and pains and wonder why. We can take a dose of our favorite analgesic, or we may find the pain and stiffness disappear after a series of stretching exercises.

Should I get a knee or hip replacement? Replacement surgery is often dictated by the severity of the pain and/or the amount of disability being experienced. Partial replacements can also be an option. Joint replacement technology constantly improves, so waiting may not be all that bad.

How soon can we realistically expect improvement from exercising? That's hard. One study said the moderately frail (however defined) showed improvement in about three months. Another study put the figure at six months. So don't get impatient; you will improve.

How long should we unsteady Seniors exercise? That's easy—the rest of our lives.

AND FROM BOTH OF US: FAREWELL!

We all want to continue to live life fully with the goal being to die young but as late as possible.

To do so, we know we must be active. We unsteady Seniors have to take charge of our lives.

It begins with our willingness to try to stay active. If that means a big change for us and even some risks, it has to be. The doctors tell us that inactivity has more risks.

Unsteady Seniors can and improve when they follow a sensible exercise program tailored to their own needs and are prudent in what they undertake. They can become more active, go for walks with friends, and get involved in other healthful and pleasant activities. Those balancing, stretchers, and strengthening exercises, done on a regular basis, pay off in wonderful dividends.

Even if an unsteady Senior like you does only half of what you find in this handbook . . .

You will steadily improve!

Always keep in mind that medical researchers tell us Seniors that unsteadiness is not the inevitable companion to aging.

And a final suggestion: We planned this handbook not to be read like a novel and then put aside. Charlie regularly uses it as a reference, and we hope you will do the same.

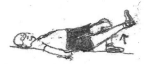

Go back and reread those sections that are relevant to your condition.

Use it to make changes in your exercise program. From time to time, check back on the exercises that Don describes. Review Charlie's stepping stones and Don's mechanisms of balance, and when you need to, check the reference section.

Few of us have perfect memories and can retain everything that we read. And sometimes when we reread, we find we missed an important point on our first run through.

Keep this handbook handy as a useful aid and watch how you as an unsteady Senior will sharply reduce the probability of falling and can live an active and satisfying life.

And so Farewell!

You now have the means to take charge of your life.

We wish you many pleasant and sunny years ahead!

Cheers!

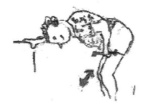

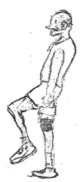

THE END

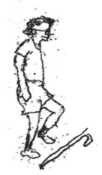

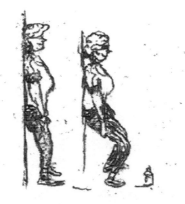

Made in the USA
Middletown, DE
13 December 2016